MRCP PART 2 EXAMINATION

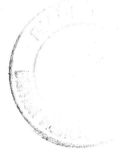

MRCP PART 2 EXAMINATION
A CANDIDATE'S REVISION NOTES

Ashley Bond MBChB

Medical Trainee, Mersey Deanery

Radcliffe Publishing
London • New York

Radcliffe Publishing Ltd
33–41 Dallington Street
London
EC1V 0BB
United Kingdom

www.radcliffepublishing.com

Electronic catalogue and worldwide online ordering facility.

British Library Cataloguing in Publication Data

A catalogue record for this book is available from the British Library.

ISBN-13: 978 1 84619 518 1

The paper used for the text pages of this book is FSC® certified. FSC (The Forest Stewardship Council®) is an international network to promote responsible management of the world's forests.

MIX
Paper from
responsible sources
FSC
www.fsc.org   FSC® C013056

Typeset by Phoenix Photosetting, Chatham, Kent, UK
Printed and bound by TJI Digital, Padstow, Cornwall, UK

Contents

Preface

This book is designed to provide MRCP candidates with a concise and well directed approach to revision; supplying a comprehensive coverage of the MRCP syllabus and the key points of each topic. Other text books have extensive text or stand alone lists. This book stands apart by supplying concise text together with the essential lists needed to pass the Part 2 exam.

The aim is not to be an extensive medical textbook, but to provide candidates with the essential knowledge required to pass the MRCP Part 2 exam. The layout is intended to facilitate effective revision in an efficient manner, as time to revise can be difficult for the modern MRCP candidate. It also provides essential guidelines from national organisations such as the British Thoracic Society and NICE.

I would like to give thanks to the contributors whose help during the process was essential.

Dr Ashley Bond
January 2011

List of contributors

Dr Stephen Pettit MBChB, MRCP, MB BS (Hons) PhD, MRCP (UK)
Specialist Registrar in Cardiology
Liverpool Heart and Chest Hospital, Liverpool.

Dr Shameena Bharucha MBChC, MRCP, MBChB, MRCP (UK)
Specialist Registrar in Gastroenterology
Royal University Liverpool Hospital, Liverpool.

Chapter 1
Cardiology

Cardiac arrhythmia
WPW
Type A:
- left sided accessory fibres
- right axis deviation
- dominant R wave in V_1.

Type B:
- right sided accessory fibres
- left axis deviation
- non-dominant R wave in V_1.

Associations:
- HOCM
- mitral valve prolapse
- Ebstein's anomaly
- secundum ASD.

Treatment – Flecanide or Amiodarone, can be used in acute phase. Ultimately ablation is gold standard. Avoid treatment with Verapamil or Digoxin, they will increase conduction down the accessory pathway and may accelerate arrhythmias.

AF and anticoagulation[1]
Paroxysmal – terminate spontaneously, lasts < 7 days.

Persistent – not self-terminating, lasts > 7 days, responds to chemical or DC cardioversion.

Permanent – continuous, does not respond to cardioversion.

CHADS2:
  C – CCF/Coronary disease = 1 point
  H – Hypertension = 1 point
  A – Age > 75 years = 1point
  D – Diabetes = 1point
  S2 – Stroke or TIA = 2 points.
0 points = aspirin.
1 point = aspirin (could consider Warfarin).
2 points = Warfarin, with an INR range of 2–3.

AF: rate versus rhythm control

Factors favouring rate control – > 65 years old:
- history of IHD.

Factors favouring rhythm control – < 65 years old:
- symptomatic
- first presentation
- correctable precipitant.

Long QT syndrome

- Due to delayed repolarisation of the ventricles.
- QT interval > 450 ms corrected in females, > 470 ms corrected in males.
- Caused by defect in alpha-subunit of potassium channel, resulting in their blockade.

Causes:
- congenital – uses genetic classification LQT1-10, examples of which are:
  - Jervell-Lange-Nielsen (recessive, associated with deafness)
  - Romano-Ward (dominant, chromosome 11).
- drugs – Amiodarone, Sotalol, TCA, Chloroquine, Erythromycin, Antipsychotics, Antihistamine (if given with cP450 inhibitors)

- electrolytes – hypokalaemia, hypocalcaemia, hypomagnesaemia
- others – SAH, hypothermia, MI, myocarditis.

Treatment:
- acquired – remove precipitant give IV potassium and IV Mg
- for congenital use Beta Blockers and ICD for high risk patients
- Digoxin causes shortening of the QT interval, but not used in the treatment of LQTS.

Indications for temporary pacing
- Symptomatic/haemodynamically unstable bradycardia.
- Second degree or CHB following MI.
- Trifascicular block prior to surgery or if symptomatic.

Inferior MI may give rise to heart block as the Posterior interventricular supplies the AV node. This is not a definite indication for temporary pacing.

Bradycardia has an increased risk of asystole if:
- HR < 40 bpm
- SBP < 100 mmHg
- LV dysfunction
- ventricular arrhythmia
- Mobitz 2
- CHB
- pauses > 3 secs
- recent asystole.

Clinical features of CHB:
- syncope
- bradycardia
- wide pulse pressure
- variable intensity of S1
- cannon A waves, irregular.

Causes of prolonged PR interval
- Idiopathic.
- Hypokalaemia.
- Digoxin toxicity.
- Myotonic dystrophy.
- Aortic root abscess.
- Sarcoidosis.
- Lyme disease.

ECG and hypothermia
- LQTS.
- Bradycardia.
- First degree heart block.
- Atrial and ventricular arrhythmia.
- J wave at end of QRS complex.

Arrhythmogenic right ventricular cardiomyopathy (ARVC)
- Is the second most common cause of sudden cardiac death in the young.
- Has an autosomal dominant inheritance with variable expression.

RV myocardium is infiltrated by fibrofatty tissue, these infiltrates act as an arrhythmogenic focus, namely for VT.

Features:
- SCD and VT
- dilated RV
- T wave inversion V1–V3
- epsilon wave seen at end of QRS.

Naxos disease is an autosomal recessive variant of ARVC. Triad of ARVC, palmar keratosis and woolly hair.

Brugada syndrome

- Autosomal dominant.
- Associated with SCD.
- Predominant in Asian population.
- Mutation in *SCN5A* gene – results in faulty Na channels.

ECG:

- convex ST elevation in V1–V3
- partial RBBB
- ECG changes absent at rest may be unmasked by sodium channel blockers, e.g. Flecainidine, Ajmaline.

Multifocal atrial tachycardia

- Is an irregular cardiac rhythm caused by at least three different sites within the atria. Each QRS complex is preceded by a p wave, however the p waves are of different morphologies and the PR intervals vary.

Most common in the elderly and those with COPD.

Treatment:

- correct any hypoxia as much as possible
- Verapamil or Beta Blockers
- Digoxin and DC cardioversion are not effective.

BP response with ETT

Normal:

- raise in systolic BP
- diastolic BP remains the same or may fall slightly.

Abnormal responses seen in hypertrophic cardiomyopathy that may indicate risk of SCD:

- fall in BP
- failure of SBP to rise
- excessive rise in SBP, e.g. > 250 mmHg.

If these responses are seen with HOCM etc then ICD insertion should be considered as the risk of SCD is high.

Heyde's syndrome

- Combination of microcytic anaemia and aortic stenosis. Commonly see angiodysplasia, the diagnosis of which is via mesenteric angiogram.
- The mechanism of bleeding is thought to arise through the destruction of von Willebrand factor, as the blood flows over the stenosed aortic valve. A combination of vWF deficiency and angiodysplasia can result in GI bleeding.
- Can see resolution of Heyde's syndrome with Aortic valve replacement.

Premature ventricular ectopics (PVE)

For a PVE to be significant they must:

- occur frequently, i.e. > 6/min
- occur in a bigeminal rhythm
- be associated with non-sustained VT
- be with R-on-T
- be associated with structural heart disease or LV dysfunction.

Broad complex tachycardia

Features that suggest VT rather than SVT with aberrant conduction:

- AV dissociation
- capture beats –intermittent conduction
- QRS concordance in the chest leads
- left axis deviation
- history of IHD
- no response to Adenosine or carotid sinus massage
- QRS > 160 ms.

Infective endocarditis

Aortic valve most commonly affected, Tricuspid most commonly affected in IVDU.

- *Strep. viridians* – mouth organism, most common organism involved.
- *Staph. aureus* – most common organism seen in IVDUs.
- *Staph. epidermidis* – most likely if < 2 months post prosthetic valve surgery.
- *Strep. bovis* – associated with carcinoma of the bowel.

Duke's criteria used in the diagnosis of infective endocarditis, diagnostic criteria:

i   pathological evidence
ii   2 major criteria
iii   1 major and 3 minor criteria
iv   5 minor criteria.

Major:
- 2 positive blood cultures for common organisms
- 3 positive blood cultures for less common organisms
- persistent bacteraemia for > 12 hours
- echo evidence of vegetation
- serology or molecular assay positive markers.

Minor:
- predisposing valve disease or IVDU
- fever > 38 degrees
- vascular phenomena
- immunological phenomena
- increase ESR or CRP.

N.B: patients with suspected IE on a prosthetic valve, initial blind therapy is Vancomycin, Rifampicin and Gentamicin.

Congenital heart disease

Transposition of the Great Arteries is the most common cyanotic lesion seen in the neonate, i.e. first few days. Overall Fallots is the most common cyanotic lesion, usually presenting at 1–2 months.

Turners (45X0) is associated with Bicuspid aortic valve (most commonly) and coarctation.

HCM (hypertrophic cardiomyopathy)
- Most common cause of sudden cardiac death.
- Due to defect in genes coding for one of the sarcomere proteins, including myosin, troponin, tropomyosin and actin.
- Autosomal dominant.
- Jerky pulse with large a wave.
- Ejection systolic murmur – increased by valsalva, standing, GTN and digoxin – decreased by squatting and Beta Blockers.

Associated with WPW and Friedreich's ataxia.

- The most useful way to assess sudden cardiac death is an abnormal BP reading during exercise tolerance testing.
- Others are positive family history, non-sustained VT, syncope, young age and increased septal wall thickness.

ECG changes:
- AF
- progressive t wave inversion in chest leads
- LVH
- deep q waves.

Fibromuscular dysplasia
- Autosomal dominant.
- Fibrous thickening of the arterial walls.
- Affects coronary, carotid and renal arteries.
- String of beads appearance seen on angiogram.
- Ultimately leads to reduced perfusion of the end organ.

Reduced renal perfusion $\longrightarrow$ activation of Renin-angiotensin system $\longrightarrow$ salt and fluid retention $\longrightarrow$ hypertension $\longrightarrow$ therefore treat with ACE-inhibitors.

Primary pulmonary artery hypertension (PAH)

Diagnosis:
- PA pressure of > 25 mmHg at rest or > 30 mmHg after exercise.

Features:
- most commonly present with exertional dyspnoea
- loud P2
- left parasternal heave – RVH
- large a waves – TR
- syncope.

Acute vasodilator testing used to determine most appropriate treatment. Patients given IV Epoprostenol or inhaled nitric oxide:
- positive test, i.e. fall in pressure – treat with calcium channel blockers
- negative test, i.e. no pressure change.

Treatment:
- Sildenafil
- Prostocyclin analogue – Iloprost
- Endothelin antagonist – Bosentan.

Aortic stenosis

If patient young, consider bicuspid valve. If older patient then calcification.

- Symptoms govern AVR – Syncope, Angina, Dyspnoea.
- If causing LV dysfunction consider AVR.
- Aortic gradient > 50 mmHg represents severe AS.

Features of severe AS:

- gradient > 50 mmHg
- quiet S2
- thrill, slow rising pulse, narrow pulse pressure
- S4
- LVH and LV dysfunction.

Supraventricular aortic stenosis – associated with William's syndrome:

- gene deletion on chromosome 7
- elfin features
- reduced mental function.

Jugular venous waveform

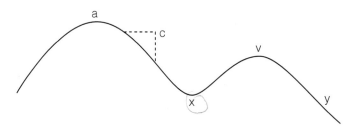

a atrial contraction (p wave on ECG)
c closure of tricuspid valve
x downward motion of heart during ventricular systole
v passive filling of atria
y filling of right ventricle through open tricuspid valve

Figure 1.1 Jugular venous waveform

Kussmaul's sign – elevation of JVP with respiration, seen in constrictive pericarditis.

Pulsus paradoxus – drop in SBP > 10 mmHg with inspiration

Table 1.1 Characteristics of jugular waveform in tamponade and constrictive pericarditis

	Tamponade	*Constrictive pericarditis*
JVP	No Y descent	X and Y descent present
Pulsus paradoxus	Present	Absent
Kussmaul's sign	Rare	Common
Other	-	Calcific lesions on CXR

Cardiac axis

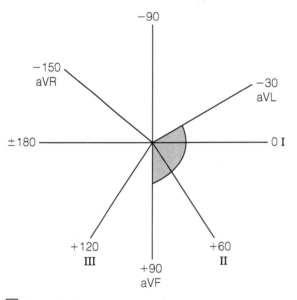

☐ Normal axis

Figure 1.2 Cardiac axis

Normal: –30 to +90.

Right axis deviation: +90 to +180.

Causes:

- PE
- RVH
- cor pulmonale

- left posterior hemi-block
- normal in infants < 1 year old
- WPW type A
- ASD, VSD, i.e. increased right out flow.

Left axis deviation: –30 to –90.

Causes:
- left anterior hemi-block
- hyperkalaemia
- WPW type B
- atrial pacing
- emphysema.

Aortic dissection

Type A – ascending aorta, proximal to left subclavian.

Type B – descending aorta, distal to left subclavian.

Initial treatment with IV Labetelol to control BP. Type A immediate surgery (mortality 1%/hr for first 48 hours). Type B can be managed medically.

Associations:
- bicuspid aortic valve (most common)
- Marfan's, Turner's
- hypertension
- pregnancy
- syphilis.

B-type natriuretic peptide

- Released from left ventricular myocardium in response to strain, i.e. HTN, CCF, valve disease, IHD, coarctation.

- Has good negative predictive value, useful prognostic indicator.
- Can be used to assess effectiveness of treatment.
- Raised levels can be due to reduced renal excretion.
- Concentrations < 100 pg/mL – unlikely to be CCF.
- Actions:
  - vasodilator
  - diuretics
  - reduced actions of renin-angiotensin system.

Myocardial action potential

Table 1.2 Myocardial action potential

Phase	Description	Mechanism
0	Rapid depolarisation	Rapid Na^+ influx
1	Early repolarisation	Efflux of K^+
2	Plateau	Slow influx of Calcium
3	Final repolarisation	Efflux K^+
4	Restoration	Na^+/K^+ ATPase

Heart sounds

S1:

- closure of mitral and tricuspid valve
- loud in mitral stenosis with opening snap.

S2:

- closure of aortic and pulmonary valves
- loud in hypertension
- soft in severe AS
- fixed splitting with ASD
- reversed split with LBBB.

S3:

- caused by diastolic filling of the ventricle, therefore increased with overloading, i.e. CCF and constrictive pericarditis

- gallop rhythm in LVF
- heard after S2.

S4:

- caused by atrial contraction against a stiff ventricle
- heard just before S1
- correlates to the p wave on ECG.

Mitral valve prolapse

Associations:

- ASD, VSD
- Cardiomyopathy
- Turner's
- Marfan's, Fragile X
- Psuedoxanthoma elasticum
- LQTS
- WPW
- Osteogenesis imperfect.

Atrial myxoma

- Is the most common cardiac tumour, 75% found within the left atrium.
- Most common in females and a cause of digital clubbing.

Features:

- left atrial dilatation
- fever, weight loss, clubbing
- mid-diastolic murmur (tumour plop)
- AF
- Emboli.

ECG and coronary territories

Table 1.3 ECG leads and coronary territories

Territory	Lead	Vessel
Anteroseptal	V1–V4	LAD
Inferior	II, III, aVF	RCA
Anterolateral	I, aVL, V4–V6	LAD OR LCx
Lateral	I, aVL, +/– V5–V6	LCx
Posterior tall r waves	V1–V2	LCx and RCA

Chapter reviewed and contributed to by Dr Stephen Pettit, MB BS (Hons), PhD, MRCP (UK), of the Liverpool Heart and Chest Hospital, Liverpool.

Chapter 2

Respiratory

Classification of acute asthma[2]

- Moderate:
  - increase in symptoms
  - PEFR 50–75%.
- Acute severe:
  - PEFR 33–50%
  - RR > 25 and HR > 110
  - inability to complete sentences.
- Life threatening:
  - PEFR < 33%
  - pO_2 < 8KPa
  - Sats < 92%
  - normal pCO_2
  - silent chest, exhaustion
  - bradycardia.
- Near fatal:
  - rising pCO_2.

Asthma stepwise treatment[2]

- Once the diagnosis of asthma has been established a stepwise treatment programme is to be adopted.
- A patient can go up and down the scale depending on their symptoms.

1 Short acting Beta 2 agonist.
2 Addition of inhaled steroid 200 mcg–800 mcg per day.
3 Addition of long acting beta 2 agonist (LABA).
4 Increase steroid to 2000 mcg per day or, Montelukast or, Oral theophylline.
5 Oral steroids.

Respiratory investigations

Spirometry

- FEV_1 – volume expired in the first second of forced expiration.
- FVC – total volume expired in forced expiration.
- FEV_1/FVC – normal = 70–80%.

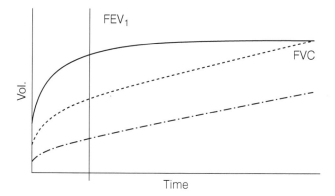

------- Obstructive- reduction in FEV_1 with a preserved FVC, i.e. asthma, COPD, bronchiectasis and bronchiolitis obliterans.

—·—·— Restrictive- reduction in FEV_1 and FVC, therefore the ration is preserved, i.e. fibrosis, asbestosis, sarcoidosis, neuromuscular disease and kyphoscoliosis.

Figure 2.1 Diagram representing spirometry

Pulmonary flow loops

- Pressure dependent collapse – as expiration begins there is an abrupt early fall, i.e. emphysema.

- Volume dependent collapse – progressive airway collapse with expiration, i.e. COPD.
- Inspiratory loop – seen if the lungs are abnormally stiff.
- Expiratory loop – if extra-thoracic obstruction exists both the inspiratory and expiratory loops of flattened, i.e. goitre.

Gas transfer

- Expressed as either DLCO or KCO, measures the transfer of CO across the alveoli.
- Raised – asthma, pulmonary haemorrhage, left to right shunt, polycythaemia.
- Low – all other respiratory diseases.

Sarcoidosis

- Granulomatous disease with giant multinucleated cells.
- 90% have thoracic involvement, therefore CXR is a vital investigation.
- CXR staging:
  0 – CXR clear
  1 – bilateral hilar lymphadenopathy (BHL)
  2 – bilateral hilar lymphadenopathy with infiltrates
  3 – diffuse pulmonary infiltrates
  4 – pulmonary fibrosis.

Features:
- most commonly asymptomatic
- dry cough
- fever and malaise
- weight loss
- raised serum ACE, ESR and Calcium
- restrictive lung pattern and reduced KCO.

HRCT findings – asymmetrical hilar lymphadenopathy, traction bronchiectasis, with perivascular septal and pleural beading.

Treatment:
- steroids
- immunosuppressants, i.e. Aziathioprine, Methatrexate.

Indications for treatment:
- parenchymal lung disease
- hypercalcaemia
- lupus pernio
- neurological and/or cardiac involvement.

Extrapulmonary manifestations:
- hepatomegaly and splenomegaly
- skin – erythaema nodosum, lupus pernio
- anterior uveitis
- neurosarcoidosis
- cardiac involvement – BBB, CHB, cardiomyopathy
- Heerfordt-Waldenstrom syndrome – parotid enlargement, uveitis, fever, cranial nerve palsy
- Löfgren's syndrome – BHL, polyarthritis, erythaema nodosum.

Occupational lung disease

Pneumoconiosis
- Due to coal dust deposition in the lung parenchyma.
- CXR diagnosis with multiple small round opacities, usually upper lobe and may cavitate.

Features:
- cough
- dyspnoea
- sputum production
- may see coal deposition within the skin
- can progress to progressive massive fibrosis – see larger opacities.

Silicosis

Due to inhalation of silicon dioxide – common in quarrying.

Features:

- acute illness, with dry cough and dyspnoea within a few months of large volume exposure
- chronic exposure results in silicate nodules, 3–5 mm in upper lobes on CXR
- eggshell calcification around hilar
- restrictive spirometry pattern, with reduced gas transfer
- compensation can be awarded.

Berylliosis

- Due to inhalation of fumes from molten beryllium.
- Result in non-caseating granulomata.

Features:

- CXR shows fine nodulation throughout fields with BHL
- positive testing with beryllium lymphocyte proliferation assay.

Byssinosis

- Due to cotton dust exposure.
- Symptoms worse on first day back at work after a break. These comprise of cough, dyspnoea, wheeze and chest tightness.
- See decline in FEV_1 over the course of the working week.

Extrinsic allergic alveolitis (EAA)

Type 3 hypersensitivity reaction towards inhaled allergen.

IgG mediated.

- Farmer's lung – *Micropolyspora faeni*.
- Bird fancier's lung – avian serum proteins, present in faeces.
- Bagassosis – *Thermoactinomyes sacchari* (sugar cane workers).

- Malt worker's lung – *Aspergillus clavatus*.
- Mushroom worker's lung – *Thermophilic actinomycetes*.

Features:
- several hours after exposure
- flu-like illness, fever, headache, myalgia
- bi-basal crepitations
- resolve within 48 hours of exposure
- chronic exposure may lead to fibrosis.

Lung fibrosis

- Upper lobe:
  - EAA
  - pneumoconiosis
  - silicosis
  - sarcoidosis
  - ankylosing spondylitis
  - TB
  - histocytosis.
- Lower lobe:
  - drugs – Methatrexate, Amiodarone
  - CFA
  - asbestosis.

Cavitating lung disease

- Squamous cell lung carcinoma.
- *Staph. aureus* pneumonia.
- TB.
- *Klebsiella* pneumonia.
- PCP.
- Rheumatoid lung disease.
- Pulmonary infarct and PE.
- Wegener's granulomatosis.

- Aspergillosis.
- Histoplasmosis.

Churg-Strauss

- A necrotising vasculitis, associated with an eosinophilia of > 10%.
- Patients will have a history of asthma.
- See sinusitis/rhinitis with mononeuritis multiplex, in combination with pulmonary disease. Together with vasculitis skin lesions.
- Eosinophilic infiltration and granuloma infiltration of affected tissue.

Investigations:
- pANCA positive
- non-fixed pulmonary infiltrates on CXR.

Treated with oral steroids.

Aspergillus and lung disease

Five main conditions seen:
1   asthma (type 1 hypersensitivity)
2   allergic bronchopulmonary aspergillosis (ABPA, type 3 hypersensitivity)
3   aspergilloma
4   invasive aspergillosis
5   EAA (malt worker's lung).

Allergic bronchopulmonary aspergillosis (ABPA)

- Most commonly seen in asthmatic patients, however can occur in non-asthmatics.
- Due to hypersensitivity to aspergillus fumigate spores.
- Mediated by IgE and IgG, therefore see raised

immunoglobulins in serum. Seventy per cent will have positive RAST testing.

Features:
- eosinophilia
- productive cough
- fleeting CXR changes
- positive skin prick testing
- positive haematoxylin and eosin (H+E) staining of sputum
- can result in bronchiectasis.

Treatment – steroids and antifungals.

Invasive aspergillosis
- Seen in patients who are immunosuppressed, a semi-invasive variant can be seen in those with mild immunosuppression, i.e. diabetes.

Features:
- fever
- cough
- dyspnoea
- pleuritic chest pain
- H+E positive staining
- focal upper lobe CXR changes.

Aspergilloma
- Cavitating lung lesion, commonly upper lobes.
- Presents with haemoptysis.
- Requires surgical removal.

Lung neoplasia
Small cell lung cancer paraneoplastic syndromes
- SIADH.
- Ectopic ACTH production (Cushing's).

- Lambert Eaton syndrome – antibodies towards Voltage Gated Calcium channels, MG like presentation.
- Peripheral neuropathy – neuronal nuclear antibody (Hu antibody).

Squamous cell lung cancer paraneoplastic syndromes
- Hyperparathyroidism.
- Gynaecomastia.
- Digital clubbing.
- Hypertrophic pulmonary osteoarthropathy – commonly affects wrists.

Adverse prognostic factors in small cell lung cancer
Factors:
- sodium < 132 mmol/l
- weight loss > 10%
- performance status > 2
- Alk phos > 1.5 times the upper limit
- LDH > 1.5 times the upper limit.

Contraindications to surgery in lung cancer
- Stage IIIb/IV.
- FEV_1 < 1.5 lit.
- Malignant effusion.
- Tumour adjacent/involving hilum.
- SVCO.
- Vocal cord paralysis.

Mesothilioma
- Most are associated with asbestos exposure, however may follow prior radiotherapy exposure. Blue asbestos most potent.
- Latent period of approximately 30 years following asbestos exposure.
- Can affect visceral and parietal pleura.

- Three histological types:
  - mixed
  - sarcomatous – worst prognosis
  - epithelial.
- Any form of biopsy gives a risk of tracking, therefore typically followed by radiotherapy.
- Spreads to the mediastinal structures.

Bronchial carcinoid

- Originate from Kulchitsky cells (neuroendocrine cells).
- Slow growing tumours, that typically occur in middle-aged adults, male = female.
- Not linked to smoking.
- Typically present with haemoptysis, may see Carcinoid syndrome.

Histology:
- occasional nuclear pleomorphism
- absent mitoses and no necrosis.

Can be associated with neuroendocrine complications, e.g. acromegaly.

Infection of the lungs

Legionella pneumonia

Incubation period of 2–10 days.

Features:
- headache, myalgia
- diarrhoea and vomiting
- abnormal LFTs
- hyponatraemia
- hypoalbuminaemia
- lymphopaenia.

Complications:
- pericarditis
- encephalitis
- renal failure.

Mycoplasma pneumonia
- Typically seen in young adults.
- Epidemics classically occur every 4 years.

Features:
- long prodrome of flu-like illness
- WCC may be normal
- bilateral consolidation.

Complications:
- haemolytic anaemia (cold agglutins IgM)
- erythaema multiforme and erythaema nodosum
- glomerulonephritis
- GBS
- DIC
- hepatitis and pancreatitis.

Poor prognostic indicators in pneumonia[3]
Confusion.
Urea – > 7 mmol/l.
Respiratory rate – > 30 per minute.
Blood pressure – systolic BP < 90 mmHg, diastolic BP < 60 mmHg.
65 – greater than 65 years old.

A point is allocated for each positive finding, those scoring > 2 classed as severe.

Other poor markers:
- bilateral lobar involvement
- pO_2 < 8 Kpa
- albumin < 35 Kpa

- WCC < 4 or > 20
- new AF.

Side effects of anti-TB drugs
- Rifampicin, Isoniazid, Pyrazinamide – hepatitis.
- Isoniazid, Ethambutol – optic neuritis.
- Isoniazid – peripheral neuropathy.
- Pyrazinamide – sideroblastic anaemia, avoid in chronic liver disease.
- Rifampicin, Isoniazid – Vit D deficiency.
- Ethambutol – colour blindness.

Must assess acetylator status prior to commencing Isoniazid, if a fast acetylator then have increased risk of hepatitis.

COPD severity

FEV_1 can be used to indicate severity of disease:
- mild 50–80%
- moderate 30–49%
- severe < 30%.

Once FEV_1 is < 50% consider high dose inhaled steroid, this is aimed at reducing exacerbation rate.

Indications for LTOT in respiratory disease

- Has been shown to reduce mortality and morbidity rates.
- Apply when patient is free of infection and other exacerbating factors.

Indications:
- pO_2 < 7.3 Kpa, or
- pO_2 < 8 Kpa with:
  - pulmonary hypertension
  - peripheral oedema
  - polycythaemia.
- FEV_1 < 1.5 litres.

Positive effects of LTOT:
- reduced mortality
- reduction in secondary polycythaemia
- reduced sympathetic outflow
- reduced cardiac arrhythmia
- improves sleep quality.

Pulmonary alveolar proteinosis (PAP)

- Alveolar sacs become filled with protein rich fluid, this can be primary or secondary to PCP, dust inhalation or haematological malignancy.
- Sputum stains positive for PAS (a protein derived from surfactant).

Features:
- PAS positive biopsy
- increase in surfactant A and D
- HRCT shows dense infiltrates and crazy paving pattern
- restrictive pattern, reduced lung capacity and reduced gas transfer.

Treated with bronchial washouts.

Lymphangioleiomyomatosis

- Most commonly affects females of reproductive years.
- Due to infiltration of immature smooth muscle cells into bronchiolar and alveolar walls. This infiltration leads to the destruction of the walls and cyst formation.
- As a result see recurrent pneumothraces and chylorous effusions.
- If seen in a male consider tuberous sclerosis as an underlying diagnosis.

Causes of bronchiectasis

- Post-infective – TB, measles, pneumonia.
- CF.
- Airway obstruction, i.e. tumour.
- ABPA.
- Sarcoidosis.
- Immune deficiency – IgA, hypogammaglobinaemia.
- Kartagener's and Young's syndrome.
- Yellow nail syndrome.

Alveolar microlithiasis

- A rare familial condition, with recessive inheritance.
- See deposits of calcium at the lung hilum and lower lobes.
- As a result of this deposition there is progressive lung disease with a restrictive pattern.
- No treatment is available, therefore supportive treatment is the only option.

Management of pneumothorax[4]

- Primary (i.e. no co-existing lung disease):
  - < 2 cm and asymptomatic – consider discharge
  - greater than 2 cm consider aspiration, if this fails intercostal drain insertion required.
- Secondary (i.e. with co-existing lung disease):
  - if patient > 50 years of age and > 2 cm in size – intercostal chest drain.

Ultrasound assistance is not required for intercostal drain insertion in pneumothorax.

Obstructive sleep apnoea

- During sleep muscle tone is reduced, the airways narrow and obstruction between the soft palate and base of the tongue occurs.
- There is poor sleep quality with daytime somnolence. Driving can be restricted.
- Obesity is the major cause, others include hypothyroidism, acromegaly, Cushing's and retrognathia.

Diagnosis is via a sleep study.

Features:
- desaturation < 90%
- tachycardia
- arousal from sleep
- cessation of airflow at the nose
- increase in oesophageal pressure swing.

Is associated with an increase in stroke.

Treatment:
- weight loss
- correct any underlying cause
- noctural CPAP, via nasal mask.

Chapter 3

Gastroenterology

Primary biliary cirrhosis

- Autoimmune disease, most commonly seen in middle-aged women.
- Most likely to present with itching or with incidental abnormal LFTs.
- There is interlobular bile duct damage due to autoimmune response, this leads to fibrosis and ultimately cirrhosis. Both of which contribute to cholestasis.

Strongly associated with other autoimmune disease, e.g. CREST, Sjögrens (seen in 80% of patients with PBC) and rheumatoid arthritis.

Features:
- raised Alk phos
- jaundice and itching
- xanthelasmata
- hyperpigmentation of the skin
- digital clubbing
- portal hypertension – hepatosplenomegaly
- increased risk of HCC (20 fold).

Diagnosis/investigations:
- raised Alk phos
- AMA positive
- raised IgM
- USS/MRCP ruled out obstruction
- positive liver biopsy.

Treatment:

- is aimed at symptom control, Ursodeoxycholic acid can be used to reduce cholestasis
- Vitamin A and D supplementation required
- ultimately liver transplantation is required.

Indications for transplant:

- Bilirubin > 100 mmol/l
- recurrent bacterial cholangitis
- ascites
- refractory itching.

Haemochromatosis

- Autosomal recessive inheritance.
- Fault found on gene coding for transmembrane glycoprotein, located on chromosome 6.
- Results in iron accumulation in parenchymal cells – i.e. liver, heart and gonads. This iron accumulation leads to end organ damage/failure.
- Affects males at an earlier age due to menstrual blood loss in females.

Features:

- usually over 40 years of age
- bronze skin pigmentation
- DM (bronze diabetes)
- abnormal LFTS, can lead to cirrhosis
- testicular atrophy
- cardiomyopathy
- chondrocalcinosis of joints on X-ray.

Diagnosis/investigations:

- raised Ferritin and Transferrin saturations
- reduced TIBC

- liver biopsy positive with Perls stain
- HFE genetic testing.

Treatment:
- venesection at regular intervals – aim for Transferrin < 50% and Ferritin < 50 mmol/l
- chelation therapy with Desferrioxamine
- screening of first degree relatives
- transplant (liver).

Cardiomyopathy and testicular atrophy can resolve with effective treatment.

Gilbert's disease

- Autosomal recessive inheritance.
- Causes a defect in conjugation of bilirubin. There is a deficiency of UDP glucoronyl transferase, as a result there is a rise in unconjugated bilirubin. Therefore not seen in the urine.
- A relatively benign condition.
- See hyperbilirubinaemia with fasting or concurrent viral illness.

Wilson's disease

- Autosomal recessive inheritance.
- Defective gene for transporting P-type adenosine triphopshate, on chromosome 13. This results in abnormal intra-hepatic production of Caeruloplasmin. As a result there is inadequate binding of copper in the biliary system, copper is therefore not excreted and accumulates. Its accumulation causes end organ damage.

Features:
- 10–25 years of age

- hepatic accumulation leads to hepatitis and ultimately cirrhosis
- Kayser-Fleischer corneal rings
- hypoparathyroidism
- neuro – reduced cognitive function, seizures, parkinsonism, tremor, chorea
- blue nails
- Fanconi's syndrome.

Diagnosis/investigation:
- reduced serum Caeruloplasmin
- increased 24 hour copper in the urine.

Treatment:
- chelation therapy with 1.5 g/day D-penicillamine.

Kings College Hospital's criteria for liver transplant in paracetamol overdose

- pH < 7.3 24 hours after ingestion of overdose.
- Or all three of:
  - PT > 100 secs
  - creatinine > 300 mmol/l
  - encephalopathy of III or more.

Causes of encephalopathy – (HEPATICUS):
Hypoglycaemia
Electrolyte disturbance
Protein meal (GI bleed)
Alcohol/analgesia
Tumour (hepatoma)
Infection
Constipation
Uraemia
Surgery.

Autoimmune hepatitis

Most common in females.

Three main subtypes, characterised by the circulating antibody:
- Type 1 – ANA +/– SMA positive.
- Type 2 – anti liver/kidney microsomal antibody (LKM1), seen in children.
- Type 3 – soluble liver-kidney antibody.

Features:
- signs of chronic liver disease
- acute hepatitis
- amenorrhoea
- raised IgG and appropriate auto-antibody.

Treatment:
- immunosuppression – steroids and steroid sparing agents
- can be considered for transplant.

Dubin–Johnson syndrome

- Benign autosomal recessive disorder.
- Due to defect in cMOAT, as a result there is defective hepatic excretion of conjugated bilirubin.
- Therefore see hyperbilirubinaemia and bilirubin present in the urine.
- Liver biopsy shows dark granules (melanin) within the hepatocytes.

Intestinal polypoid related syndromes
FAP Coli
- Autosomal dominant.
- Mutation in APC tumour suppressing gene on chromosome 5.
- Colonic malignancy inevitable, often at 30–40 years of age.

Extracolonic manifestation:
- retinal pigment hypertrophy
- fibromas
- epidermoid cyst
- supernumerary teeth.

Hereditary non-polyposis colorectal cancer (HNPCC)
- Autosomal dominant inheritance.
- Abnormality on chromosome 2.
- Amsterdam criteria used for diagnosis.
- Associated with increase in breast, endometrial and ovarian malignancy, along with colonic.

Cowden syndrome
- Hamartomatous polyposis syndrome.
- Defect in PTEN tumour suppressor gene.
- See polyp formation in GI tract, oral cavity and along nasal mucosa.
- Increased risk of malignancy, especially breast and thyroid.
- Can have thyroid dysfunction even post thyroidectomy.

Gardener's syndrome
Autosomal dominant condition.

Features:
- multiple adenomatous intestinal polyps
- osteomas
- soft tissue tumours, i.e. fibromas, lipomas.

Ninety per cent will develop bowel carcinoma by the age of 45 years.

Colectomy recommended once polyps appear.

Peutz–Jegher's syndrome
- Autosomal dominant.

- Characterised by numerous hamartomatous polyps in GI tract.
- Typically see pigmented freckles around lips, face, palms of hands and soles of feet.
- Increased incidence of GI bleed and intussusceptions.
- Approximately 50% will die from GI cancer before the age of 60.

Coeliac disease

- Gluten sensitivity enteropathy, arises from a sensitivity to the gliadin fraction of wheat. This sensitivity evokes an autoimmune response that results in villous atrophy in the proximal small bowel.
- Ninety-five per cent are HLA DQ2 positive.

Associations:
- dermatitis herpetiformis
- type 1 diabetes
- autoimmune hepatitis
- PBC
- autoimmune thyroid disease
- positive family history
- IBS.

Features:
- diarrhoea
- cramping abdominal pain
- weight loss
- oral ulcers
- general malaise
- anaemia
- malabsorption
- digital clubbing
- 50% can have positive faecal occult blood.

Small bowel biopsy – crypt hypertrophy, lymphocyte infiltration and villous atrophy.

Diagnosis/investigation:
- positive antibodies
- Antiendomysial (can be negative if IgM low)
- Antigliadin
- tissue transglutaminase.

Complications:
- Folate, B_{12} and iron deficiency
- increase in all GI malignancy, especially GI lymphoma
- hyposlenism – see target cells and Howell-Jolly RBCs on film
- osteomalacia
- subfertility.

Treatment:
- avoidance of gluten containing foods, i.e. rye, wheat, oats and barley
- if a gluten free diet is adhered to then villous atrophy can resolve.

Causes of villous atrophy:
- Coeliac disease
- Tropical sprue
- Whipple's disease
- lymphoma
- hypogammaglobinaemia
- giardia
- lactose intolerance.

Whipple's disease

- Caused by *Tropheryma whippelli* infection.
- Most common in HLA-B27 positive people and middle-aged men.

- Jejunal biopsy see macrophages containing Periodic acid-Schiff (PAS) granules.

Features:
- malabsorption and weight loss
- large joint arthralgia
- lymphadenopathy
- hyperpigmentation and photosensitivity
- digital clubbing
- neuro – ataxia, myoclonus, seizures, dementia.

Treatment:
- 6–12 months of Ampicillin.

MALT lymphoma (mucosa-associated lymphoid tissue)

- Associated with *H. pylori* in 90% of cases.
- Most commonly seen in the stomach.
- If low grade than 80% will respond to eradication of *H. pylori* alone.

Other *H. pylori* associated GI disease:
- DU (95%)
- gastric carcinoma
- atrophic gastritis.

VIPoma (vasoactive intestinal peptide)

- VIP is released from small bowel and pancreas. It acts to increase pancreatic and small bowel secretions and to reduce acid production.

Features:
- 90% arise from pancreas
- large volume diarrhoea

- weight loss
- hypokalaemia, hypochloraemia
- achlorhydria – reduced gastric acid
- raised plasma chromogranin A.

Zollinger-Ellison and multiple endocrine neoplasia (MEN)

- Zollinger-Ellison disease arises from a Gastrin secreting tumour that arises from the duodenum or pancreas. It results in large volume acid secretion, gastric irritation and ulceration.
- Typically presents with epigastric pain and diarrhoea.
- 30% occur as part of MEN.

Diagnosis:
- can be achieved with Secretin test, positive if gastrin level > 200 pg/mL.

Table 3.1 Multiple endocrine neoplasia

MEN I	MEN IIa	MEN IIb
Chromosome 11	Chromosome 10	Chromosome 10
Tumours – parathyroid	Tumours – parathyroid	Tumours – parathyroid
• Pancreas	• Phaeochromocytoma	• Phaeochromocytoma
• Pituitary	• Medullary thyroid	• Medullary thyroid
		• Marfanoid
		• Mucosal neuromas

Inflammatory bowel disease
Crohn's disease

- Can affect any part of the GI tract. Most commonly affects the terminal ileum, colon and anorectum.
- Transmural inflammation, histologically see non-caseating granulomata.
- Abdominal pain and frequent fever prominent.

Associations:
- increased incidence in smokers
- skin erythaema nodosum, pyoderma gangrenosum
- irisits/uveitis
- arthritides, sacroilitis
- cholelithiasis
- digital clubbing.

Diagnosis/investigations:
- barium studies:
  - cobblestoning
  - skip lesions
  - rosethorn ulcers
  - strictures.

Anti-*Saccharomyces cerevisiae* antibody positive.

Complications:
- fistulae
- abscess formation
- malabsorption
- increased risk of carcinoma.

Ulcerative colitis
- Rectum almost always involved, with disease extending backwards into colon.
- Continuous lesion. Terminal ileum can be affected by 'backwash' ileitis. Rest of gut unaffected.
- Only mucosa and submucosa affected.
- Bloody diarrhoea predominates.

Associations:
- reduced incidence in smokers
- increased incidence of:
  - PBC

- primary sclerosing cholangitis
- chronic active hepatitis.
- other systemic manifestations occur, but less commonly than in Crohn's.

Diagnosis/investigations:
- barium studies:
  - featureless bowel
  - pseudopolyps.
- colonoscopy and biopsy
- pANCA positive.

Complications:
- large increase in carcinoma
- malabsorption
- acute exacerbation with megacolon.

Assessing the severity of UC exacerbation – the following can be used to say the exacerbation is severe:
- > 6 bloody stools per day
- ESR > 30
- HR > 90
- pyrexia
- anaemia.

Risk of GI carcinoma in inflammatory bowel disease
The risk of developing malignancy as a direct result of IBD is increased if:
- onset at < 15 years of age
- disease duration > 10 years
- total colitis
- disease with unremitting course
- poor treatment compliance.

Budd–Chiari syndrome

Due to thrombotic or non-thrombotic obstruction of the hepatic venous flow.

Consists of a triad of:
- abdominal pain
- tender hepatomegaly
- ascites.

Therefore can be seen in any prothrombotic state, i.e. SLE, Antiphospholipid syndrome, OCP, pregnancy and Behçet's.

Treatment is with anticoagulation.

Oesophageal motility disorder

Can be assessed by symptoms and manometry.

- Scleroderma – see low lower-oesophageal resting pressure.
- Spasm – see raised lower-oesophageal resting pressure.
- Achalasis – absence of distal peristalsis. Also see rat-tail pattern on barium swallow.

Melanosis coli

- Is a disorder of pigmentation of the bowel wall.
- Pigment laden macrophages are seen on biopsy.
- It is associated with laxative abuse, specifically Senna.

Viral hepatitis

Hepatitis A
- RNA virus.
- Spread via faeco–oral route.
- Causes anorexia, jaundice, joint pains, fever, nausea and vomiting.

- Self-limiting disease with no chronicity.
- Treatment is supportive only.
- Vaccine available.

Hepatitis B

- DNA virus.
- Spread via blood, sexual contact and vertically.
- Acutely causes fever, arthritis, glomerulonephritis, arteritis.
- Can result in fulminate failure.
- 5% chronicity rate.
- Vaccine available.

Hepatitis C

- RNA virus.
- Spread via blood and sexual contact.
- Causes acute hepatitis.
- 85% chronicity rate.
- Increased risk of HCC.
- No vaccine available.

Hepatitis D

- Incomplete virus.
- Blood borne transmission.
- Relies on concurrent Hep B infection.
- Increased incidence of cirrhosis when co-infects with Hep B.

Hepatitis E

- RNA virus.
- Spread via faeco–oral route.
- Acute self-limiting disease.
- Treatment is supportive.
- Can be serious if infection occurs in pregnancy, leading to fetal and/or maternal mortality.

Chapter 4
Infectious disease and GUM

Infections and tropical disease
Malaria
- Protozoa infection of the red blood cells.
- Transmitted by female mosquito.
- Four types seen:
  1 *Plasmodium falciparum*
  2 *Plasmodium vivax*
  3 *Plasmodium ovalae*
  4 *Plasmodium malariae*.
- *Falciparum* has the potential to be the most severe.
- *Vivax* and *ovalae* can lay dormant in the liver for some time.
- Diagnosis is via giemsa thick-and-thin films. Thick will tell the presence of a protozoa and the thin film will type it.

Severe *Falciparum* malaria:
- markers of severity:
  - parasite count > 1%
  - temperature of > 39°C
  - schizonts on blood film
  - hypoglycaemia
  - severe anaemia.
- complications:
  - cerebral malaria – seizures, coma, hypertonia, hyperreflexia, nystagmus, papilloedema

- acute renal failure – black water fever (due to widespread intravascular haemolysis)
        - ARDS
        - DIC
        - hypoglycaemia
        - splenic rupture.

- Treatment:
        - if not severe/complicated oral quinine can be used
        - severe or complicated use IV quinine
        - if suspect resistance add Doxycycline
        - non-falciparum treat with Chloroquine.

Schistosomiasis

- Is a parasitic flat worm infection.
- There are three principal species:
        - *S. mansoni* and *japanicum* (affect liver and bowel)
        - *S. haematobium* (affect urinary tract).
- Acquired from fresh water, i.e. swimming.
- *Mansonia* and *japanicum* are found in the venous plexus of the portal tract, whilst *haematobium* is found in the bladder.
- They release a large number of eggs, these pass into the liver or bladder wall. As a result there is inflammation and ultimately can see fibrosis, i.e. hepatic fibrosis or obstructive uropathy. May see urinary frequency, haematuria or calcification.
- Increased risk of future bladder cancer.

Treatment – Praziquantel.

Leishmaniasis

Caused by the intracellular protozoa *Leishmania*, usually spread by sand flies.

Three main forms are seen:

1   cutaneous:
     – due to *Leishmania tropica, mexicana*
     – crusted lesion at the site of sand fly bite
     – underlying ulcer to the lesion.

2   mucocutaneous:
     – caused by *Leishmania brasiliensis*
     – skip lesions may spread to involve the nose and pharynx.

3   visceral:
     – common in India, incubation period of 2–8 months
     – due to *Leishmania donovani*
     – fever, rigors, sweats
     – massive hepatosplenomegaly
     – pancytopaenia
     – grey skin discolouration.

Treatment is complex and best undertaken in specialist units.

Measles

- Due to a RNA paramyxovirus.
- Spread via respiratory droplet, with incubation period of 10–14 days.
- The host is infective from the start of the prodrome until five days after the rash has appeared.

Features:

- prodrome of irritability, conjunctivitis and fever
- rash – maculopapular rash, classically begins around the ears and spread to rest of body becoming confluent
- Koplik spots – white spots within the mouth, seen on buccal mucosa.

Complications:

- Pneumonia – most immediate
- Encephalitis – seen 1–2 weeks after infection

- subacute sclerosing panencephalitis – can be seen years later, rare
- myocarditis
- increase in appendicitis
- diarrhoea

Leptospirosis (Weil's disease)

- Due to spirochete *Leptospira interrogans*.
- Spread via rat urine, therefore common in sewage worker, farmer, vets or abattoir workers.
- Can be contracted from swimming in water where rats have been, i.e. canals.

Features:

- fever
- flu-like illness
- renal failure (up to 50%)
- hepatic dysfunction and jaundice
- subconjunctival haemorrhage
- meningitis and headache.

Treatment – Benzylpenicillin or Doxycycline.

Tetanus

- Caused by Tetanospasmin exotoxins released from *Clostridium tetani*.
- Found in the soil.
- Tetanospasmin prevents the release of GABA.

Features:

- Prodrome – fever, lethargy, headache
- trismus (lock-jaw)
- risus-sardonicus – facial spasm that produces a grin
- opisthotonus – arched back and hyperextended neck
- dysphagia due to oesophageal spasm.

Treatment:
- Metronidazole
- may require ventilatory support and muscle relaxants
- tetanus Ig for high risk wounds.

Chagas disease (American Trypanosomiasis)
- Due to protozoan *Trypanosoma cruzi*.
- Spread by Tsetse fly.
- See acute and chronic disease.

1   Acute – 95% are asymptomatic, the remainder will see an erythematous nodule at the site of the bite or periorbital oedema.

2   Chronic disease affects the bowel and heart. It can result in megacolon or megaoesophagus, thus resulting in perforation. Also may see myocarditis, leading to cardiomyoapthy and death from failure and arrhythmia. Cardiac involvement is the most common cause of death.

Diagnosis via thick and thin films.

Treatment – Nifurtimox.

African Trypanosomiasis
- Due to *Trypanosoma brucei rhodesience*.
- Again transmitted by tsetse fly.

Features:
- Initially erythema at bite site, then
  - headache
  - insomnia
  - daytime sleeping and behavioural change
  - coma (sleeping sickness).

Diagnosis – CT head, LP and thick/thin films.

Treatment – Nifurtimox.

Typhoid
- Typhoid and parathyphoid are caused by *Salmonella typhi* and *Salmonella paratyphi* (types A, B and C).
- Gram-negative rods, aerobic, not normally found in the gut.
- Normally termed enteric fevers.
- Persistent fever in a tropical traveller, and malaria excluded, think Typhoid.
- Do not have to have diarrhoea and vomiting.

Features:
- week 1 – pyrexia, inappropriate bradycardia and constipation
- week 2 – maculopapular rash (rose spots), lymphadenopathy, hepatosplenomegaly
- week 3 – complications: pneumonia, endocarditis, osteomyelitis, haemolytic anaemia, meningitis, GI bleed.

Diagnosis achieved via positive culture of bacteria, i.e. stool, blood.

Treatment – Cephalosporin or Quinalones.

Toxoplasmosis
- Due to the protozoa, *Toxoplasma gondii*.
- Infects via the GI tract, lungs and broken skin.
- Commonly affects eyes, brain and muscle.
- Most infections are asymptomatic and usually self-limiting.
- Most significant in the immunosuppressed, i.e. HIV.
- Common reservoir is the domestic cat and their faeces.

Features:
- resembles EBV – fever, malaise, lymphadenopathy
- meningoencephalitis

- cerebral abscess
- myocarditis.

Congenital toxoplasmosis:
- due to transplacental spread from the mother
- results in microcephaly, hydrocephalus, cerebral calcification.

Diagnosis – achieved with positive antibody testing and Sabin-Feldman dye test.

Treatment – Pyrimethamine and Sulphadiazine.

Cholera
- Due to the bacteria *Vibrio cholerae*, a Gram-negative bacillus.
- Short incubation period of 24–48 hours.
- Upon infection it acts to stimulate Adenylate cyclase within the bowel, this results in chloride excretion, causing large volume osmotic diarrhoea.

Features:
- painless, large volume 'rice water' diarrhoea, faint fishy smell
- later see abdominal pain
- severe dehydration – resulting in death
- people of O blood group at increased risk.

Treatment:
- primarily aim to adequately hydrate
- antibiotics are used to limit spread rather than as a direct treatment. Those used are Doxycycline, Ciprofloxacin, Erythromycin.

Lyme disease
- Tick borne disease, due to infection with *Borrelia burgdorferi*.
- Most common tick borne disease in northern hemisphere, seen after walking in long grass.

Early features:

- erythema migrans
- fever
- malaise
- arthralgia.

Late features:

- heart block
- cranial nerve palsy
- meningitis
- polyarthitis.

Treatment – Doxycycline and Benzylpenicillin.

Diphtheria

- Due to Gram positive, *Corynebacterium diphtheria*.
- Common in Eastern Europe.
- Humans are the common reservoir, transmitted person to person via contact.

Features:

- exudative pharyngitis, with soft tissue swelling and lymphadenitis – Bull neck
- may affect skin, eyes and genitalia
- the exotoxins can cause myocarditis and neuropathy.

Treatment is supportive, but antibiotics such as Erythromycin can be used to eliminate transmission/carriage.

Dengue fever

- Due to arthropod-borne *Flavivirus*.
- Incubation period of 7 days.

Features:

- fever
- retro-orbital pain

- maculopapular rash
- myalgia
- haemorrhagic fever-bleeding, lymphocytosis.

Treatment – supportive.

Tick typhus
- Due to infection with *Rickettsia conorii*, Gram negative cocci.
- Commonly seen after walking in South African scrublands.

Features:
- fever
- headache
- lymphadenopathy
- bite marks and localised erythema.

Treatment – exclude malaria, Doxycycline.

Brucellosis
- Infection with *Brucella spp*, a Gram negative rod.
- Acquired via unpasturised milk or from close contact with cattle.

Features:
- insidious onset, fever, headache, myalgia and sweats
- bone pain
- bradycardia
- splenomegaly
- deranged LFT's
- leukoerythroblastic picture on blood film.

Diagnosis:
- blood cultures
- serum agglutin testing
- bone marrow biopsy.

Treatment – Doxycycline and Rifampicin.

Rocky Mountain spotted fever

- Infection with tick-borne *Rickettsia rickettsii*.
- Seen in those visiting North America, will give history of tick bite.

Features:

- maculopapular rash, commonly starting at wrists and ankles, then spreading to the rest of the body
- also affects palms of hands and soles of feet.

Treatment – Doxycycline.

Strongyloidiasis

- A soil dwelling worm, common in Africa and Southeast Asia.
- Transmission is via larval penetration of the soles of feet when walking barefoot on soil.

Features:

- diarrhoea
- abdominal pain
- larva currens rash (serpiginous)
- solid organ abscesses.

Risk is dramatically increased in immunocompromised people.

Treatment – Ivermectin.

Yaws

- Caused by *Treponema pertenue*, therefore VDRL and TPHA positive.
- Transmitted via skin to skin contact.

Features:
- multiple wart like lesions, these may break down and form ulcers
- hyperkeratosis of palms of hands and soles of feet.

Diagnosis – via Dark field microscopy.

Treatment – IM penicillin.

HIV and related disease
HIV life cycle
Is a retrovirus, with a tropism for CD4 cells.

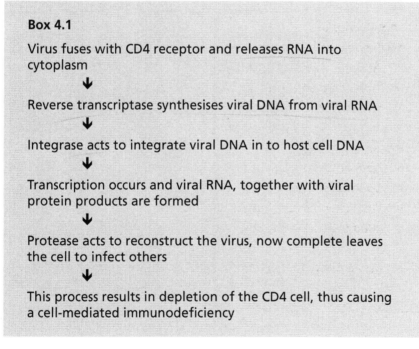

Box 4.1

Virus fuses with CD4 receptor and releases RNA into cytoplasm
↓
Reverse transcriptase synthesises viral DNA from viral RNA
↓
Integrase acts to integrate viral DNA in to host cell DNA
↓
Transcription occurs and viral RNA, together with viral protein products are formed
↓
Protease acts to reconstruct the virus, now complete leaves the cell to infect others
↓
This process results in depletion of the CD4 cell, thus causing a cell-mediated immunodeficiency

Diagnosis:
- incubation period of 2–4 weeks following infection
- it can take up to 3 months before HIV 1 and 2 antibodies are detectable

- one-third of patients will develop a seroconversion illness, during this illness HIV PCR and p24 antigen testing can confirm the diagnosis.

Seroconversion features:
- are very non-specific, and mimic many other conditions, therefore should have high index of suspicion
- macular rash, fever, lymphadenopathy
- headache, photophobia
- diarrhoea
- arthralgia
- meningio-encephalitis.

Is usually self-limiting lasting approximately three weeks.

Markers of disease progression:
- falling CD4 count, normal – > 500, AIDS defined when < 200
- high viral load
- polyclonal gammopathy
- increase Beta 2 microglobulin
- increased neopterin
- development of AIDS defining disease, e.g. PCP, oesophageal candidiasis.

HIV treatment:
- typically started when CD4 count falls below 350
- the two main targets for treatment are Reverse transcriptase and Proteases.

1   Reverse transcriptase:
- nucleoside reverse transcriptase inhibitors (NRTI), e.g. Zidovudine, Lamivudine, Stavudine
- non-nucleoside reverse transcriptase inhibitors (NNRTI), e.g. Nevirapine, Efavirenz.

2   Protease inhibitors (PI), e.g. Indinavir, Atazanavir.

The combination of these is known as HAART (Highly Active Anti-Retroviral Therapy), e.g. combination of two NRTI and one of a NNRTI or PI.

Side effects:
- NRTI:
  - all: lipoatrophy, lactic acidosis and cardiomyopathy
  - Zidovudine: myopathy, anaemia, marrow toxicity, nail changes.
- NNRTI – interact with cP450s:
  - Nevirapine = Hepatitis
  - Efavirez = hallucination and vivid dreams.
- PI – all:
  - lipoatrophy, diabetes, hypertriglycerideaemia, buffalo hump, central adiposity, cP450 inhibitor
  - Indinavir: renal calculi
  - Atazanavir: hyperbilirubinaemia (mimics Gilbert's disease).

HIV/AIDS related diseases

1 *Pneumocystis carinii* pneumonia (PCP):
- due to pulmonary infection with the fungus *Pneumocystis jiroveci*
- classed as an AIDS defining illness.

Features:
- dry cough
- fever
- oxygen desaturation with exercise
- lymphadenopathy
- hepatosplenomegaly
- CXR – bilateral interstitial shadowing (can be normal).

Diagnosis – positive culture from sputum/bronchoalveolar lavage.

Treatment:

- those with low CD4 count can have prophylactic treatment with oral Co-Trimoxazole or Nebulised Pentamidine
- active infection treated with Co-Trimoxazole, severe cases with IV Pentamidine
- those with hypoxia benefit from the addition of steroids, e.g. $pO_2 < 9.3$ KPa.

2 Progressive multifocal leucoencephalopathy (PML):

- caused by infection with JC virus, may indicate a CD4 count < 100
- CT shows white matter lesions that are non-enhancing, with no midline shift or surrounding oedema
- enhancing lesions on CT head are seen in toxoplasmotic abscesses and cerebral lymphoma
- JC virus positive PCR from LP sample also diagnostic.

Other HIV related CSF analysis:

- HHV8 PCR – positive in Kaposi sarcoma
- CMV and HHV-encephalitis
- EBV PCR – primary cerebral lymphoma.

3 CMV retinitis:

- can be slowly progressive or sudden, with retinal haemorrhage and detachment
- patients will describe reduced visual acuity
- a sight threatening condition.

Treatment:

- IV Ganciclovir + HAART
- if there is evidence of marrow suppression then substitute Ganciclovir for Foscarnet.

4 HIV and diarrhoea:

- can be due to the virus itself, i.e. HIV enteritis or opportunistic infection.

Cryptosporidium:
- an intracellular protozoa
- incubation period of 7 days
- modified ZN stain used for diagnosis, via stool sample.

Treatment is usually supportive, can consider Nitazoxamide.

Mycobacterium avium intracellulae:
- an atypical *mycobacterium*, usually seen when CD4 count < 50.

Features:
- fever
- abdominal pain
- sweats
- diarrhoea
- hepatomegaly and hepatic dysfunction
- marrow infiltration.

Treatment:
- Rifampicin
- Ethambutol
- Clarithromycin.

Genital ulceration

- Painful – herpes >> chancroid.
- Painless – syphilis > lymphogranuloma venereum and granuloma inguinale.

1 Lymphogranuloma venereum:
- due to infection with *Chlamydia trachomatis*
- occurs in three stages:
  - i   painless pustules that then form painless ulcers
  - ii   painful inguinal lymphadenopathy
  - iii proctocolitis.

2   Granuloma inguinale:
- due to infection with *Klebsiella granulomatis*
- results in multiple painless genital ulcers.

3   Chancroid:
- due to infection with *Haemophilus ducreyi*
- common in Caribbean, Africa and South West Asia.

Features:
- painful genital ulcers
- lymphadenopathy
- 'school of fish' Gram-negative rods on culture.

Treatment –Azithromycin or Ciprofloxacin.

Classification of bacteria

- Gram negative cocci – *Neisseria meningitidis* (diplococcus), *Neisseria gonnorrhoeae*.
- Gram negative bacillus – *Haemophilus influenzae*.

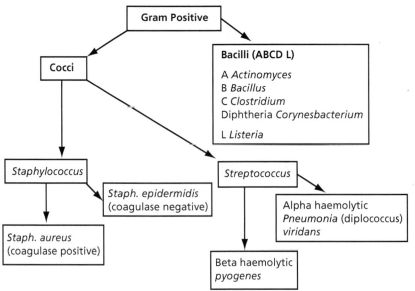

Figure 4.1 Classification of bacteria

Infective diarrhoea

- *E. coli* – incubation period of 12–48 hours:
  - commonest form of diarrhoea in a traveller
  - watery stools
  - nausea, vomiting and abdominal cramps
  - 0157 associated with Haemolytic Uraemic syndrome.
- *Shigella* – incubation period of 48–72 hours:
  - result is bloody diarrhoea
  - highly contagious
  - nausea, vomiting and abdominal pain.
- *Campylobacter* – 48–72 hours incubation period:
  - flu-like prodrome with fever
  - diarrhoea may be bloody, associated with abdominal pain
  - complications include GBS and reactive arthritis.
- *Staph. aureus* – incubation 1–12 hours:
  - enterotoxins cause severe vomiting.
- *Giardia* – spread via faeco–oral route:
  - incubation period of > 7 days
  - infection can be asymptomatic
  - prolonged diarrhoea and steatorrhoea
  - treated with Metronidazole.

Meningitis

Table 4.1 CSF findings in meningitis

	Bacterial	Viral	TB
Appearance	cloudy	Clear/cloudy	Fibrin web
Glucose	< 50% of serum	Normal	< 50% of serum
Protein	> 1 g/L	Normal	> 1 g/L
WCC	polymorphs	lymphocytes	lymphocytes

Gram staining of CSF and bacterial associations:
- *Staph. epidermidis* – is associated with the presence of a VP shunt

- *Strep. pneumoniae* – a Gram-positive diplococcus
- *N. meningitides* – a Gram-negative diplococcus
- *H. influenza* – Gram-negative bacillus
- *Listeria monocytogenes* – small Gram-positive bacillus, associated with unpasteurised soft cheese.

Vaccinations

Live attenuated (therefore pose a risk in immunocompromised patients):
- BCG
- yellow fever
- MMR
- oral polio
- oral typhoid.

Whole killed organism:
- pertussis
- rabies.

Fragment:
- Diphtheria
- Tetanus
- Meningococcus, pneumococcus, haemophilus.

Chapter 5

Pharmacology and toxicology

Overdose and poisoning

Lead poisoning

- Lead can accumulate within the body via various routes, e.g. ingestion, inhalation, through skin. If food is contaminated, such as fish from lakes polluted with lead, toxic levels can be seen.

Features:
- lethargy
- renal failure
- hypertension
- microcytic anaemia
- peripheral neuropathy (motor)
- constipation
- hearing loss
- blue discolouration of gum margins.

Treatment – chelation therapy with Dimercaptosuccinic acid.

Lithium toxicity

- This can be both unintentional and intentional.
- Adequate levels monitoring requires 12-hour post dose levels.

Causes:
- intentional

- dehydration
- drugs – diuretics, ACE-inhibitors, NSAIDs, Phenytoin, Tetracyclins, Ciclosporin.

Features:
- coarse tremor
- confusion
- thirst
- seizure
- coma.

Treatment – stop lithium, fluid resuscitation, can consider haemodialysis.

Acute dystonia
- Can be seen following use of Haloperidol, Metoclopramide and Phenothiazides.
- May present as oculogyric crisis – fixed lateral flexion of neck, fixed deviation of eyes, profuse sweating and lacrimation.

Treatment – Procyclidine.

Organophosphate poisoning
- Can be unintentional, commonly seen in those working in agriculture.
- Results in acetylcholinesterase inhibition, therefore see accumulation of acetylcholine and excessive stimulation of cholinergic system.

Features (SLUD):
- **S**alivation
- **L**acrimation
- **U**rination
- **D**efecation
- bradycardia

- hypotension
- miosis
- muscle paralysis, leading to death.

Treatment:
- removal all clothing and washing skin thoroughly
- IV atropine
- Pralidoxime.

Beta Blocker

- Treatment not always required immediately, it will depend upon amount taken and haemodynamic stability.
- If bradycardic and hypotensive, or large dose taken treat with high-dose glucagon.
- Potassium closely monitored as can rise significantly in overdose.
- May have to consider temporary pacing.

Methanol toxicity

- Methanol is metabolised by alcohol dehydrogenase to formaldehyde and formic acid, these products are toxic. Resulting in metabolic acidosis, blindness and death within 30 hours of significant ingestion.

Features:
- increased anion gap
- visual impairment
- seizures
- fundoscopy – hyperaemic disc, engorged veins, papilloedema.

Treatment:
- IV Ethanol or Fomepizole – compete for alcohol dehydrogenase
- IV bicarbonate
- dialysis can be used to remove methanol.

Methaemoglobinaemia
- Results from the oxidation of Fe^{2+} to Fe^{3+} within the haemoglobin of red blood cells. In this state the haemoglobin cannot carry oxygen, therefore inducing a functional anaemia.

Causes:
- Primaquinine
- Trimethoprim
- Sulphonamide
- Lidocaine
- Metoclopramide
- Dapsone.

Features:
- dyspnoea, headache, dizziness
- seizures
- chocolate cyanosis (nails, lips and ears)
- normal oxygen saturations and low pO_2.

Treatment – methhaemoglobin can be measured on ABG, if > 20% then give Methylene Blue, otherwise stop the offending drug and observe.

Neuroleptic malignant syndrome
- Can be seen following the use of antipsychotics and dopamine antagonist, e.g. Metoclopramide and Haloperidol.

Features:
- whole body rigidity
- pyrexia
- extrapyramidal signs
- elevated CK and AST.

Treatment:
- IV fluids

- Bromocriptine
- Dantrolene.

Theophylline overdose

Features:
- hypokalaemia
- seizures
- hyperglycaemia
- hypercalcaemia
- confusion.

Treatment:
- if present within 2 hours of overdose repeated activated charcoal and gastric lavage can be used
- seizures controlled with diazepam/lorazepam
- charcoal haemoperfusion
- propanolol can be given if potassium low and have tachycardia, however not in asthma.

Antidepressant overdose

1 Tricyclics:
- potentially life threatening, mainly due to cardiac arrhythmia.

Features:
- anticholinergic – blurred vision, dry mouth, urinary retention, constipation
- Long QT, may lead to VT
- seizures and coma.

Treatment:
- IV sodium bicarbonate, in a less acidic environment the TCA binding to proteins increases, therefore reducing its bioavailability.

2 SSRIs:
- an overdose state results in Serotonin Syndrome.

Features:

- restlessness
- hallucinations
- hyperthermia
- ataxia
- hyperreflexia
- dilated pupils
- tachycardia
- myoclonus.

Cyanide poisoning

May be seen following smoke inhalation, i.e. in a house fire.

Features:

- in large doses will quickly lead to death
- dyspnoea and hyperventilation
- tightness in the chest
- pre-syncope.

Treatment:

- dicobalt edetate
- sodium thiosulphate
- sodium nitrate.

Paraquat poisoning

- Is a pesticide, will follow intentional ingestion.
- Ingestion of > 10 g carries 100% mortality, death usually results from pulmonary fibrosis in the second week following ingestion.
- A plasma level of > 0.1 g/mL carries a poor prognosis.

Treatment:

- gastric lavage if present within 6 hours of ingestion
- Fullers Earth and activated charcoal may also be used.

Aspirin overdose

- As time elapses following an overdose a pattern of symptoms and signs will evolve. Initially the patient will hyperventilate, resulting in a respiratory alkalosis. At this point they may all describe tinnitus.
- As time passes their acid-base status will alter to a metabolic acidosis, resulting in severe vomiting and hypokalaemia. If this continues untreated coma and death may result.

Treatment:
- IV fluids
- charcoal if present early enough
- IV sodium bicarbonate
- replace potassium
- haemodialysis.

Indication for dialysis:
- severe acidosis
- hepatic or renal dysfunction
- pulmonary oedema
- salicylate level > 700 mg/l.

Iron overdose

- Serum iron levels can be used to assess severity and therefore prognosis, a level of > 90 mmol/l suggest a severe overdose and carries a poor prognosis.

Features:
- diarrhoea and vomiting
- dark stool
- abdominal pain
- AXR may show tablets within the bowel.

Treatment:
- if present within one hour of ingestion activated charcoal
- whole bowel Klean-prep

- IV desferrioxamine
- IV fluids.

Interaction and important side effects

Drug induced gynaecomastia

- Omeprazole.
- Cimetidine.
- Spironolactone.
- Amiloride.
- Finasteride.
- Digoxin.
- TCA.

Drugs to avoid in G-6-PD deficiency

- Primaquine.
- Nitrofruantoin.
- Quinalones.
- Sulphonamides.

Drugs to avoid in porphyria

- Erythromycin.
- Cephalosporins.
- Diclofenac.
- TCAs.
- MAOIs.
- Antihistamines.
- Simvastatin.
- Sodium valproate.

Drug induced urticaria

- Aspirin.
- NSAIDs.
- Penicillins.
- ACE-inhibitors.

- Thiazides.
- Codeine.

Drug Induced gum hypertrophy
- Amlodipine.
- Phenytoin.
- Ciclosporin.
- Nifedipine.

Drug induced hyperprolactinaemia
- Metoclopramide.
- Domperidone.
- Haloperidol.
- Phenothiazides.
- SSRIs.

Drug induced photosensitivity
- Amiodarone.
- Bendroflumethiazide.
- Ciprofloxacin.

Drug induced impaired glucose tolerance
- Thiazides.
- Steroids.
- Tacrolimus.
- Ciclosporin.
- Interferon alpha.
- Nicotinic acid.
- Antipsycotics.

Drug induced psoriasis
- Lithium.
- Beta blockers.
- Antimalarials.
- NSAIDs.

Bisphosphanates and osteonecrosis of the jaw

- Caused by nitrogen containing bisphosphanates, e.g. Zolendronic acid.
- Results from the anti-resorptive action of the drug.

Features:
- deep ulceration and jaw pain.

cP450 inhibitors and inducers

1 Inducers – i.e. reduce the effectiveness of other drugs, e.g. OCP, Warfarin. Carbamazepine is a self inducer:
- Phenytoin
- Carbamazepine
- barbiturates
- Rifampicin
- alcohol (chronic)
- St John Wort
- sulphonylureas.

2 Inhibitors – i.e. increase the effect of other drugs, e.g. Warfarin, Theophylline:
- Omeprazole
- Metronidazole
- Disulfiram
- Erythromycin
- Valproate
- Isoniazid
- Ciprofloaxacin, Cimetidine, cranberry juice
- ethanol (acute)
- sulphonamides.

Drug conversions

1 Opiates:
- Morphine to Oxycodone – divide by 2

- Codeine to Morphine – divide by 10
- Morphine to SC Diamorphine – divide by 3
- Morphine to Fentanyl patch – 90 mg = 25 mcg/hr
- Breakthrough, divide total 24-hour dosing by 6.

2 Steroids:
- 1 mg Prednisalone = 4 mg Hydrocortisone
- 1 mg Dexamethasone = 7 mg Prednisalone.

Dopamine and its actions

- At different flow rates Dopamine has distinct actions, via different receptor sites.
- 0.5–2 mcg/Kg/min – D_1 and D_2, leading to increased mesenteric and renal blood flow.
- > 2 mcg/Kg/min – $Beta_1$ receptors, causing increased HR and myocardial contractility.
- > 10 mcg/Kg/min – $Beta_1$, $Alpha_1$ and $Alpha_2$, resulting in renal vasoconstriction and reduced renal blood flow.

Doxapram

- Is a respiratory stimulant that can be considered in those who are unable to tolerate NIV.
- Usually given at a rate of 1–4 mg/min.
- Half-life of 3–4 hours.

Contraindications:
- IHD
- epilepsy
- hyperthyroidism
- stroke
- phaeochromocytoma.

Side effects:
- hypertension
- agitation – especially in those patients on theophylline
- headache
- nausea and vomiting.

Chapter 6
Ophthalmology

Acute red eye

1 Acute angle closure glaucoma:
- symptoms are worse when the pupil is dilated, typically worse at night
- halos described around lights
- severe pain, associated with nausea and vomiting, occasionally with abdominal pain
- semi-dilated, non-reactive, oval shaped pupil, with hazy cornea
- associated with hypermetropia
- sight threatening.

Treatment – topical Pilocarpin and IV Acetazolamide.

2 Anterior uveitis/iritis:
- painful loss of vision
- blurred vision, associated with photophobia
- small, fixed pupil with ciliary flush
- associated with systemic disease e.g. IBD, Ankylosing Spondylitis, reactive arthritis and Behçet's?

3 Episcleritis:
- severely painful red eye
- pain worse on movement, tender nodularity to the sclera
- should consider an underlying autoimmune condition.

4 Subconjunctival haemorrhage:
- non-sight threatening
- self-limiting and benign.

Pupillary disorders

See Chapter 9 for further notes.

Horner's syndrome
Caused by damage to the sympathetic innervations of the eye and surrounding structures.

Features:
- Ptosis
- Miosis
- Anhidrosis (absence of sweating)
- Enopthalmus
- congenital Horner's leads to a difference between the two colours of the iris (heterochromia).

The Anhidrosis can be used to determine the site of the underlying lesion:
- head, arm and trunk – central lesion (stroke, Syringomyelia, MS, tumour)
- just face – pre-ganglionic (Pancoast tumour, trauma, thyroidectomy)
- absent – post-ganglionic (cavernous sinus thrombosis, cluster headache, carotid artery dissection, carotid aneurysm).

Holmes-Adie's pupil
- Benign condition, more common in females.
- Causes dilation of the pupil, 80% are unilateral.
- Patients have a hypersensitivity to Pilocarpine.
- Associated with a loss of deep tendon reflexes.
- Once the pupil does constrict it is slow to recover.

Ectopia lentis

Describes subluxation of the lens.

Associated with:
- Homocystinuria – inferior displacement
- Marfan's – superotemporal displacement
- Ehlers-Danlos
- Refsum's disease
- Weill-Marchesani (patients are of short stature).

Ophthalmological association with systemic disease

Retinitis pigmentosa
- Progressive inherited disease that affects the photoreceptors and retinal pigment epithelium.

Consists of a triad of:
- night blindness
- tunnel vision
- pigmented bony spicule on fundi.

Important associations:
- Abetalipoproteinaemia
- Kearns-Sayre syndrome – mitochondrial inheritance, see first-degree heart block
- Refsum's disease
- Usher's syndrome
- Alport's syndrome.

Sickle cell anaemia
- Associated with Black Sunburst picture on the retina.
- This is pathognomonic of SCA.

Bear track retina
- Appear as small-pigmented lesions in the peripheral retina of both eyes. Is formally known as congenital hypertrophy of retinal pigment epithelium.
- Is strongly associated with FAP, therefore if seen patients should be referred for investigation of large bowel.

Angioid retinal streaks
- Appear as irregular dark red streaks on the retina.
- Associated with:
  - Paget's disease
  - SCA
  - Acromegaly
  - Ehlers-Danlos syndrome
  - Pseudoxanthoma elasticum.

Optic atrophy
- Pale well demarcated disc on fundoscopy.
- Usually bilateral.

Causes:
- acquired:
  - smoking
  - methanol
  - MS
  - chronic papilloedema
  - glaucoma
  - ischaemia
  - B_1, B_2, B_6, B_{12} deficiency.
- congenital:
  - Friedreich's ataxia
  - Wolfram's syndrome
  - Leber's optic atrophy.

Retinopathy

Macular degeneration
- Most common cause of blindness in the UK.
- Due to degeneration of the central retina.

Risk factors:
- > 60 years old

- female
- positive family history
- smoking
- caucasian.

Two types:
1 dry – characterised by yellow Drusen spots
2 wet – see neovascularisation, carries worst prognosis.

Treatment:
- stop smoking
- high dose Beta-carotene, Vit C and E and Zinc (must stop smoking prior)
- wet – laser therapy and Anti-VEGF, e.g. Ranibizumab
- dry – no cure.

Features of diabetic retinopathy

Background:
- microaneurysm
- flame and blot haemorrhage
- hard exudates.

Pre-proliferative:
- cotton wool spots (soft exudates)
- venous beading.

Proliferative:
- neovascularisation
- haemorrhage
- detachment.

Chapter 7
Renal

Glomerulonephritis (GN)

Minimal change
- Most common cause of GN in children.
- Almost always presents with Nephrotic syndrome (oedema, hypoalbuminaemia and proteinuria > 3.5 g/24 hours, may also see hypercholesterolaemia).
- Renal function may be normal.

Histology – under electronmicroscope see loss of foot processes from podocytes. May appear normal under light microscope.

Causes:
- NSAIDs
- Gold
- Hodgkin's lymphoma
- Thymoma.

Treatment – is with steroid, with this treatment the majority will resolve. But there may be intermittent future relapse.

Membranous glomerulonephritis
- Commonest type seen in adults.
- Consists of nephrotic syndrome, renal failure and asymptomatic proteinuria.

Histology – granular IgG and complement 3 deposition along the glomerular basement membrane (GBM).

Causes:

- Malignancy – colon, bronchus, stomach, CLL
- connective tissue – SLE, rheumatoid arthritis, Sjögrens
- infection – Hepatitis B+C, malaria, syphilis
- drugs – gold, NSAIDs, penicillamine
- others – Sarcoid, GBS, PBC.

Treatment:

- Heparin
- sodium restriction
- diuretics
- Ponticelli regime (steroids and Chlorambucil).

- 1/3 will progress to end stage renal failure (ESRF).
- 1/3 will respond to treatment.
- 1/3 will resolve spontaneously.

Focal segmental

- Most commonly affects middle-aged men.
- Presents with renal failure, nephrotic syndrome and proteinuria.
- Commonly leads to ESRF.
- For those who undergo renal transplantation there is a high rate of recurrence in the transplanted kidney.

Histology – deposits of IgM.

Associations:

- obesity
- IV heroin use
- HIV – in these patients should commence HARRT and ACE-inhibitors.

IgA nephropathy (mesangioproliferative, Berger's disease)

- Is a disease of young adults.

- Can be seen following URTI or sore throat.
- Twenty-five per cent will go on to develop ESRF, those whom present with haematuria are less likely to do so.

Histology – mesangial hypercellularity, IgA and C3 deposition along GBM.

Associations:
- cirrhosis
- coeliacs
- Henoch–Schönlein purpura.

Treatment –steroids are used in those who are nephritic.

Mesangiocapillary
- Patients present with nephrotic syndrome and proteinuria.
- Fifty per cent will progress to ESRF.
- See reduced C3.

Histology – double contouring of GBM.

Two types:
1 subendothelial immune deposits. Causes – cryoglobulinaemia, Hepatitis C
2 intramembranous deposits, reduced C3. Causes – partial lipodystrophy, factor H deficiency.

Diffuse proliferative
- Seen post-streptococcal infection.
- Presents with acute renal failure and nephrotic syndrome.
- Associated with reduced C3.

Histology – diffuse proliferation of cells within glomeruli.

Most will resolve spontaneously without intervention.

Rapidly progressive

- Associated with Goodpasture's and Wegener's, therefore cANCA and pANCA levels are important. Also associated with pulmonary haemorrhage.
- See rapid deterioration in renal function.
- Overall mortality around 20%.

Histology – linear deposits of IgG on basement membrane.

Treatment:
- high dose Methylprednisalone
- Cyclophosphamide
- plasmapheresis.

Renal disease and complement levels (C3 and C4)

Complement levels can be measured to aid in diagnosis prior to any renal biopsy.

Low complement associated with:
- post-streptococcal GN (diffuse proliferative)
- mesangiocapillary GN
- renal failure associated with endocarditis
- renal disease in SLE.

Renal tubular acidosis (RTA)

- There are four types of renal tubular acidosis.
- They are associated with hyperchloraemic metabolic acidosis, with a normal anion gap.

Type 1 (distal):
- associated with sickle cell anaemia
- results from an inability to excrete H^+, therefore have impaired urinary acidification

- urinary pH typically > 5.3
- plasma bicarbonate < 10 mmol/l
- hyperkalaemia.

Complications·
- nephrocalcinosis and calculi
- UTI.

Type 2 (proximal):
- due to a failure of bicarbonate resorption
- typically plasma bicarbonate 14–20 mmol/l
- serum potassium low/normal.

Complications:
- oesteomalacia
- ricketts
- Fanconi syndrome.

Renal cell carcinoma and Wilm's tumour

Renal cell carcinoma
Arises from proximal renal tubular epithelium.

Associations:
- smoking
- tuberous sclerosis
- von Hippel-Lindau syndrome.

Features:
- loin pain, palpable mass
- haematuria
- weight loss
- commonly spreads to bone, therefore bony pain and fractures
- development of a left sided varicocele, i.e. compression of left renal vein

- hormonal disorder:
  - PTH-like hormone, i.e. hypercalcaemia
  - renin secreting, leading to hypertension
  - Cushing's, due to ectopic ACTH secretion
  - Epo secreting, therefore polycythaemia.

Treatment (stage dependent) – surgery +/– interlukin-2 or Sunitinib (tyrosine kinase inhibitor).

Wilm's tumour

- Is a tumour of childhood, usually seen before five years of age.
- Derived from embryonic renal tissue.

Features:

- abdominal mass (95% are unilateral)
- haematuria
- 20% have metastases at the time of presentation, most commonly lungs.

Associations:

- Beckwith-Wiedemann syndrome
- WAGR syndrome
- Defect on chromosome 11.

Treatment is a combination of surgery, chemotherapy and radio-therapy. Treatment carries an 80% cure rate.

Polycystic kidney disease (PCKD)

Arises from a defect in polycystin protein.

- Type 1 – defect on chromosome 16 (most common).
- Type 2 – defect on chromosome 4.

Features:

- haematuria
- positive family history
- chronic renal failure, may result in ESRF and dialysis
- loin/flank pain – may present acutely if there is cyst rupture
- hypertension – best treated with ACE-inhibitors
- hypercalcaemia, hyperphosphataemia.

Associations:

- hepatic cysts
- intracranial aneurysms – may present with SAH.
- mitral valve prolapse
- polycythaemia, secondary to increase Epo.

Renal calculi

- Calcium based stones are the most common.
- Oxalate stones are commonly seen following small bowel resection.
- Urate and xanthine stones are radiolucent.
- Struvite (staghorn) stone are associated with *proteus* urinary infection.
- Cysteine stones are semi-opaque.

Causes:

- dehydration
- hypercalcaemia, i.e. hyperparathyroidism
- Cystinuria
- Type 1 renal tubular acidosis
- drugs – loop diuretics and steroids.

Renal Medullary Calcification seen in RTA Type 1, meduallary sponge and hyperparathyroidism.

Calcium related renal stones can be reduced by Thiazide diuretics.

Renal transplantation and graft rejection

The timing of any rejection indicates the type and prognosis. Immune-modulation will be required in order to control any rejection.

1 Accelerated dysfunction:
   - IgG mediated
   - seen in the first 1–5 days following transplant
   - presents with fever, pain over graft and rapidly rising creatinine.

2 Acute rejection:
   - occurs between 5 days and 3 months following transplant
   - not typically painful, but see a steadily rising creatinine
   - can be confirmed with renal biopsy
   - responds rapidly to pulsed Methylprednisalone.

3 Chronic allograft rejection:
   - seen > 3 months following transplant
   - a silent, symptomatic process
   - see uncontrolled hypertension, proteinuria and a slowly rising creatinine.

Immunotherapy options:
   - Ciclosporin – can itself cause renal failure
   - Tacrolimus – calcineurin inhibitor
   - Aziathioprine – monitor for marrow suppression
   - Mycophenalate
   - Steroids.

Renal calculations
Calculated anion gap

$$(Na^+ + K^+) - (Cl^- + HCO_3^-)$$

Normal = 8–16 mmoL

Causes of raised anion gap:
- DKA
- lactic acidosis
- renal failure
- ethylene glycol ingestion
- methanol ingestion
- aspirin overdose.

Calculated serum osmolarity

$$2(Na^+ + K^+) + Urea + Glucose$$

Important in the diagnosis of SIADH, DI and the investigation of serum sodium abnormalities.

Side effects of Epo treatment in CRF

For those who have anaemia secondary to their CRF, treatment with Epo can improve symptoms. Side effects of this treatment are:
- hypertensive crisis
- headache
- seizures
- hyperkalaemia
- thrombosis
- pure red cell aplasia
- induction of iron deficiency.

Indications for urgent dialysis/filtration in renal failure

- pH < 7.1.
- Pulmonary oedema.
- Potassium > 6.5 mmol/l or associated ECG changes.
- Uraemic pericarditis or other uraemia related symptoms.

Proteinuria and its significance

- The degree of proteinuria can be used to detect early renal disease in patients with diabetes and hypertension. It can be used as an indicator for commencing treatment, namely with ACE-inhibitors.
- Microalbuminuria – 30–300 mg/24 hours – in diabetics indicates need for ACE-inhibitors.
- Albuminuria – > 300 mg/24 hours.
- Proteinuria – > 3.5 g/24 hours.

Albumin/creatinine ratio (ACR)
- ACR is recommended by NICE to monitor CKD.
- A spot sample of the first pass morning sample is used.
- Significance differs between diabetics and non-diabetics.

Non-diabetics – > 30 mmol/l.
Diabetics – > 2.5 mmol/l, commence treatment with ACE-inhibitors.

Chapter 8

Haematology and oncology

Bleeding disorders and coagulopathy

Haemophilia

- Typically X-linked recessive, therefore more common in male.
- Some have no family history and arise from spontaneous mutations.

Two types:

1. Haemophilia A – most common, deficiency of factor VIII
2. Haemophilia B – deficiency of factor IX, also known as Christmas disease.

Features:

- severity depends on the degree of deficiency, termed severe when clotting factor measures less than 1%
- see spontaneous bleeding, classically within muscle and joints
- prolonged bleeding after injury or surgery
- see prolonged APTT, with reduced associated clotting factors
- PT and thrombin time are normal.

Treatment:

- replacement of deficient factors, this does put patients at risk of blood borne infections
- tranexamic acid.

Von Willebrand disease

- The production of vWF is coded for on chromosome 12.
- Is the most common inherited coagulopathy in the UK.
- vWF is a large glycoprotein that promotes platelet aggregation, along with acting as a carrier molecule for factor VIII.

Three types:

1. partial reduction in quantity (most common)
2. abnormal form
3. complete absence of vWF (most severe).

Features:

- manifests as platelet derived bleeding tendencies, i.e. bruising, purpura and menorrhagia
- mildly prolonged APTT (less so than will haemophilia)
- reduced levels of factor VIII
- low levels of vWF.

Treatment:

- tranexamic acid
- Desmopressin – causes an increase in release of vWF from endothelial cells
- Factor VIII replacement.

Antithrombin III deficiency

- Is a thrombophilic disorder, i.e. see increased clot formation.
- Autosomal dominant inheritance.
- Antithrombin III normally acts to inhibit the actions of Factor X, IX and thrombin, therefore its normal physiological action is to limit thrombosis. If deficient, there is excessive factor X, IX and thrombin activity leading to thrombosis.
- Heparin acts by binding with Antithrombin, therefore if see ongoing thrombosis in the presence of heparin consider Antithrombin III deficiency.

- Will most commonly present with venous thrombosis, i.e. recurrent DVT and/or PE.

Treatment – in the presence of recurrent thrombosis will be anticoagulation with Warfarin.

Factor V Leiden deficiency
- Is an inherited thrombophilia.
- If heterozygous have a milder thrombotic tendency.
- Is the most commonly inherited thrombophilia is Europe.
- The defect results in the production of Factor V Leiden that is resistant to the actions of Protein C, and therefore cannot be inactivated. As a result there is increased thrombosis.

Features:
- recurrent DVT, PE and other venous thromboses
- women of the OCP are at high risk and it should be stopped
- those who are homozygous have highest risk, heterozygous patients can be monitored prior to anticoagulation.

Protein C deficiency and Warfarin
- Protein C is produced in the liver, is a Vitamin K dependent factor and is vital in preventing thrombus formation.
- Is inherited in an autosomal dominant fashion.
- Becomes very important if Warfarin is prescribed.

Warfarin is a Vitamin K antagonist that acts via the inhibition of Vitamin K epoxide reductase. In doing so it reduces the production of clotting factors II, VII, IX and X. When initially started warfarin causes a paradoxical reduction in protein C and S, thus being pro-thrombotic. It can result in thrombosis in the skin venules causing Warfarin induced skin necrosis. Hence the used of LMWH cover in the first five days of Warfarin treatment.

Antiphospholipid syndrome

An acquired disorder.

Features:
- elevated APTT, thrombocytopaenia
- increased venous thrombosis
- recurrent miscarriage
- livedo reticularis
- adrenal infarct may causes Addisonian picture.

Treatment:
- Warfarin if have thrombosis
- aspirin during pregnancy.

Specific clotting factor deficiency

The effect of different clotting factor deficiencies can be identified through their effects on the PT and APTT.

- Factor VII – prolonged PT.
- Factors IX, VIII, XI, XII – prolonged APTT.
- Factors II, V, X – both prolonged PT and APTT.

Mixing studies with 50:50 testing can be used to distinguish between factor deficiency and the presence of inhibitors, i.e SLE, acquired Factor VIII deficiency. If the coagulopathy corrects with the 50:50 testing then it is due to clotting factor deficiency.

Thrombocytopaenia

Idiopathic thrombocytopaenia purpura (ITP)
- Is an immune mediated reduction in platelets.
- Is acquired, and commonly follows a viral infection.
- Due to autoantibodies that are directed towards Glycoprotein IIb/IIIa on the platelet surfaces.
- If platelets become severely low there is a risk of bleeding.

Features:
- acute:
  - most common in children
  - male–female
  - may follow viral infection
  - purpuric rash
  - increased bleeding tendencies
  - self-limiting.
- chronic:
  - most common in young women
  - follows a relapse-remitting course.

Can be associated with Evans syndrome when see ITP with autoimmune haemolytic anaemia.

Treatment:
- immune-modulation therapy
- steroids (first line)
- Cyclophosphamide
- IV Ig.

A splenectomy can be considered in those not responding to treatment, those with a platelet count of < 30 after three months of steroid treatment can be considered.

Thrombotic thrombocytopaenia purpura (TTP)
- A severe and life threatening condition. It carries a near 100% mortality if left untreated.
- Can occur during pregnancy or in the postpartum period.
- Results from an acquired autoantibody, the actions of this antibody produce inhibition of the enzyme ADAMTS 13. In doing so there is failure to cleave the large vWF multimers. These large multimers cause excessive platelet aggregation within small vessels. As the red blood cells pass through these abnormally narrowed vessels they are haemolysed. Therefore overall see haemolysis and thrombocytopaenia.

Features:
- confusion and fluctuating neurological signs
- pyrexia
- acute renal failure
- thrombocytopaenia
- microangiopathic haemolytic anaemia (MAHA)
- increased reticulocytes count
- death will follow if not treated.

Treatment:
- will likely require high level care
- plasma exchange.

Features of microangiopathic haemolytic anaemia:
- anaemia
- helmet cells
- reticulocytes
- fragment cells.

Haemolytic uraemic syndrome (HUS)
Most commonly seen in children, however can also affect adults.

Triad of:
- acute renal failure
- MAHA
- thrombocytopaenia.

Do not get the neurological symptoms seen in TTP.

Overall mortality can reach 10%, with the worst prognosis in adults.

Causes:
- *E. coli 0157*
- SLE
- HIV
- pregnancy.

Treatment:
- supportive
- plasma exchange.

Disseminated intravascular coagulation
- Results from a massive pro-coagulant state.
- There is large-scale activation of platelets and clotting factors, together with destruction of fibrin. Therefore see thrombosis, consumption of platelets and clotting factors, followed by haemorrhage.
- Can be acute or chronic.

Features:
- abnormal clotting
- reduced fibrinogen and raised D-dimer
- thrombocytopaenia
- MAHA
- haemorrhage
- carries a very poor prognosis.

Need to look for underlying cause, e.g. infection or malignancy. If have a leukoerythroblastic picture on blood film, i.e. immature RBC and WCC consider marrow invasion with malignant cells.

Causes:
- amniotic fluid embolus
- pre-eclampsia
- retained products of conception
- crush injury
- infection
- transfusion reaction
- malignancy.

Treatment:
- is ultimately to remove driving force, i.e. infection etc. If this is not possible then DIC will almost always result in death

- FFP, cryoprecipitate and platelets can be used to correct bleeding.

Heparin induced thrombocytopaenia (HIT)

- This describes the reduction in platelets that can be seen following treatment with Heparin.

There are two main types.

1. Type 1 – non-immune disorder. See fall in platelets within the first few days of treatment. Occurs as a result of the direct action of heparin on platelet activation. Platelets do not fall below 100 and will recover with continued treatment.

2. Type 2 – is an immune-mediated process. Typically seen five days after treatment started. Platelets fall dangerously low. Require a > 50% reduction for diagnosis. The binding of the autoantibody to the platelet causes clot formation and reduction in overall platelet count. HIT can therefore predispose to thrombosis formation, consequently there may be extension of existing thrombus or the formation of new ones.

Treatment:

- if suspected Heparin should be stopped, this includes Heparin used in line flushes
- platelet and antibody testing can be used to confirm
- Danaparoid is used for anticoagulation once heparin is stopped.

Haemolysis
Site of haemolysis

- Intravascular:
  - paroxysmal nocturnal haemoglobinuria
  - cold autoimmune haemolytic anaemia
  - red cell fragmentation, i.e. valve haemolysis

- G-6-PD deficiency
- mismatch blood transfusion.
- Extravascular:
  - haemoglobinopathies – SCA, Thalassaemia
  - hereditary spherocytosis
  - warm haemolytic anaemia
  - haemolytic disease of the newborn.

The direct Coombs' test

- A positive test will confirm the presence of haemolysis, but not the cause. Further investigation will be required once haemolysis is confirmed.
- It detects the presence of antibodies on the RBCs of a patient. These antibodies can have different functions:
  - complement fixing – thus complement derived destruction
  - opsonisation – attracting phagocytic cell
  - agglutinating – clumping of RBCs.

Paroxysmal nocturnal haemoglobinuria

- An acquired, complement induced haemolysis.
- Due to a post-translocation modification.

RBCs lack the GPI anchor protein, this absence makes them susceptible to complement driven destruction.

Features:

- haemolytic anaemia, intravascular
- may see pancytopaenia
- dark urine, haemoglobinuria, classically seen in the morning
- thrombosis, increased risk of stroke, due to lack of CD59 on platelet surface.

Diagnosis:

- Hams test can be used
- flow cytometry looking for reduced CD59 and CD55.

Treatment:

- anticoagulation
- blood product replacement when required.

Hereditary spherocytosis

- Autosomal dominant condition.
- Defect results in abnormal spectrin within the structure framework of RBCs. As a result they lose their bi-concave shape and become spherocytes. In this state they are more fragile and recognised as abnormal, therefore are lysed by the spleen (i.e. extravascular).

Features:

- haemolytic anaemia
- jaundice (pre-hepatic)
- pigment gallstones
- increased Mean corpuscular haemoglobin count
- aplastic crisis when infected with Parovirus.

Diagnosis:

- positive osmotic fragility testing
- spherocytes seen on blood film.

Treatment:

- folate replacement
- splenectomy.

Glucose-6-Phosphate dehydrogenase deficiency (G-6-PD)

- X-linked inheritance.
- Most commonly seen in Africa, Mediterranean and Middle East.
- Neonatal jaundice can occur, but most have a normal haemoglobin and blood film until crises occur.

G-6-PD provides protection to RBCs against oxidative stress, therefore in its absence, this protection is lost. Oxidative crises can be induced by:

- drugs – Primaquine, Ciprofloxacin, Sulfonamides
- infection
- Fava beans (Favism).

Features – exposure to oxidative stress, leading to rapid haemolysis, anaemia and jaundice with RBC Heinz bodies.

Treatment:
- avoid/remove precipitant
- supportive
- transfusion if required.

Autoimmune haemolytic anaemia
- Are divided into Warm and Cold, according to at what temperature haemolysis is best induced.
- Most common idiopathic.

1 Warm:
- seen at body temperature
- IgG mediated
- extravascular haemolysis.

Causes:
- SLE
- CLL
- Lymphoma
- Methyldopa.

Treatment – responds well to Prednisalone, 1 mg/kg/day.

2 Cold (paroxysmal cold haemoglobinuria):
- IgM mediated
- intravascular haemolysis.

Causes:
- mycoplasma infection

- EBV
- Lymphoma.

Treatment – does not respond as well to steroids as Warm. Can consider IV Ig.

Drug induced haemolysis
Drugs that may cause haemolysis are:
- Penicillins
- Cephalosporins
- Methyldopa
- Quinine
- NSAIDs.

Haematological malignancy
Chronic myeloid leukaemia
- Is a disease of middle age.
- Ninety-five per cent of patients have the Philadelphia translocation (9;22). This translocation results in the fusion of the ALB proto-oncogene with the BCR gene. Consequently there is increased tyrosine kinase activity and cell division.

Features:
- most present with tiredness, weight loss and sweats
- large WCC
- anaemia
- splenomegaly
- low neutrophil alkaline phosphatase score
- hyperleucocytosis leads to visual disturbance, priapism
- 80% transform to AML
- marrow biopsy shows hypercellular picture with increased myeloid precursors.

Treatment – Imatinib, monoclonal antibody, acts to inhibit tyrosine kinase, by binding to the BCR-ABL receptors.

Chronic lymphocytic leukaemia

- Due to monoclonal proliferation of well-differentiated lymphocytes, 99% of which are B cell in origin. Can be asymptomatic and found incidentally on FBC. When there is a lymphocyte count > 5×10^9, in the absence of infection.
- Most common in the elderly.

Features:
- often asymptomatic
- B cell symptoms – night sweats, weight loss, lethargy
- lymphadenopathy
- increased infection, due to hypogammaglobinaemia
- hepatosplenomegaly
- elevated LDH and Alk Phos.

Complications:
- warm haemolytic anaemia
- transformation to high-grade lymphoma
- hypogammaglobinaemia.

Investigations:
- elevated lymphocyte count on FBC
- mature looking lymphocytes and smear (smudge) cells on blood film
- CD19 and CD20 positive cells with immunophenotyping.

Indications for treatment:
- progressive marrow failure
- massive lymphadenopathy
- progressive lymphocytosis > 50% rise over two months
- systemic symptoms.

Chemotherapy with a Chlorambucil containing regime is the mainstay of treatment.

Poor prognostic factors:
- male
- over 70 years old
- lymphocyte count > 50
- elevated LDH
- positive CD38 cells
- lymphocytes doubling time < 12 months.

Acute myeloid leukaemia
- Is associated with increasing age and prior myeloproliferative disorders.
- See blast cells containing Auer rods.
- These cells stain positive for Sudan Black and Myeloperoxidase.
- Marrow biopsy shows increased cellularity of myeloid lineage.

Poor prognostic indicators:
- cytogenes showing chromosome 5 or 7 deletion
- older age
- prior marrow disease, i.e. myelodysplasia.

Treatment:
- marrow hypoplasia required to induce remission
- Arabinoside based chemotherapy
- if WCC high Leucocytopharesis is used to reduce the count. This is essential prior to blood transfusion to prevent complications of hyperviscosity.

Acute promyelocytic leukaemia
- A subtype of acute myeloid leukaemia.
- Due to the (15;17) translocation, results in the fusion of PML and RAR alpha genes.

Features:
- elevated WCC

- increased infection rates
- DIC
- Thrombocytopaenia
- younger age at presentation.

Treatment – all-trans-retinoic acid.

Hairy cell leukaemia
- Malignant proliferation of B cells.
- These B cells appear with villous projection on the blood film, giving the condition its name.
- Most common in males.

Features:
- pancytopaenia
- splenomegaly
- skin vasculitis
- dry marrow tap
- TRAP positive staining
- 'fried egg' appearance of bone marrow biopsy.

Waldenstrom's macroglobulinaemia
- Is a lymphoplasmacytoid malignancy.
- See monoclonal IgM paraprotein secretion. IgM has a large pentamer structure, as a result hyperviscosity is a major complication.

Features:
- IgM paraproteinaemia
- weight loss
- hyperviscosity – thrombosis, visual loss
- hepatosplenomegaly
- lymphadenopathy
- cryoglobulinaemia – may result in Raynaud's.

Treatment – chemotherapy based around Cyclophosphamide and Doxorubicin.

Myeloma and monoclonal gammopathy of undetermined significance (MGUS)

- Myeloma is a neoplastic proliferation of plasma cells, as a result there is large volume production of their immunoglobulins and light chains.
- Clinical manifestations are due to the excess of these substances and marrow infiltration.
- Classification is based upon the cell product, i.e. IgG (most common), IgA and light chain disease. Disease involving IgG and IgA production may also see light chain production, these appear in the urine as Bence Jones protein. They may cause significant renal damage.

Features:
- bone pain
- pathological fractures
- renal failure
- anaemia
- recurrent infection
- hyperviscosity.

Investigations:
- monoclonal proliferation of immunoglobulins
- Bence Jones protein in urine
- hypercalcaemia, raised ESR
- renal impairment
- punched out lesions on X-rays, e.g. pepper pot skull.

Diagnosis – this requires 1 major and 1 minor, or 3 minor criteria to be met.

- Major:
  - plasmacytoma on marrow biopsy

- – > 30% plasma cell on bone marrow biopsy
- – monoclonal band on electrophoresis or light chains in urine (of significant levels).
- Minor:
  - – 10–30% plasma cells on bone marrow biopsy
  - – abnormal monoclonal band, but to levels seen in major criteria
  - – immunosuppression.

Treatment:

- bisphosphanates used to control hypercalcaemia and bone pain
- adequate hydration required to protect renal function
- chemotherapy regimes
- Thalidomide
- survival is worse with declining renal function and development of anaemia.

Monoclonal gammopathy of undetermined significance (MGUS) arises when patients are found to have a paraprotein of a level that is not significant for diagnostic criteria. Along with no end organ damage, i.e. renal failure or bone involvement. Over an extended period of time the paraprotein level remains stable. It is essential that they are monitored at regular intervals as this can be a 'pre-myeloma' phase.

Burkitt's lymphoma and EBV related disease

- Is a high-grade B cell lymphoma.
- Due to *c-myc* gene translocation (8;14).

Two types:

1 endemic – commonly seen in Africa, affects mandible/maxilla. Due to infection with EBV
2 sporadic – abdominal tumours are most common, typically around ileo-caecal valve. Increased incidence in HIV positive patients.

Features:
- B cell symptoms
- lymphadenopathy
- weight loss
- marrow involvement and recurrent infection
- may see extranodal spread.

Other EBV related malignancy:
- Hodgkin's lymphoma
- nasopharyngeal carcinoma
- hairy leukoplakia
- HIV CNS lymphoma.

Hodgkin's lymphoma (HL)

- Represents malignant proliferation of lymphocytes, is separated histologically from the non-Hodgkin's lymphomas by the presence of Reed-Sternberg cells.
- Two peaks of incidence, young adults and the elderly.

Features:
- B cell symptoms – night sweats, weight loss
- alcohol induced lymph pain
- lymphadenopathy
- pruritis
- hepatosplenomegaly
- anaemia, raised LDH, urate, calcium and ESR.

The Ann Arbor Classification System is used to stage HL.
Stage I – a single lymph node area or single extranodal site.
Stage II – two or more lymph node areas on the same side of the diaphragm.
Stage III – involvement of lymph areas on both sides of the diaphragm.
Stage IV – multiple involvement of extranodal sites, i.e. liver, marrow.

With the addition of A or B.

A – no B cell symptoms.

B – presence of B cell symptoms.

Treatment options are highly dependent upon the histological type, grade and stage. It may consist of radiotherapy and/or chemotherapy. Bone marrow transplantation is an option after myeloablative therapy.

Gene translocations

- t(9;22) – Philadelphia chromosome, *BCR-ABL* gene. Seen in CML.
- t(8;14) – *c-myc* oncogene. Seen in Burkitt's lymphoma.
- t(11;14) – *cyclin-D1* gene. Seen in Mantle cell lymphoma.
- t(15;17) – *PML-RAR* alpha gene. Seen in acute promyelocytic leukaemia.

Oncological therapies

Chemotherapy agents

Table 8.1 Chemotherapy agents, mode of action and common side effects

Drug	Mode of Action	Side effects
Vincristine	Inhibits the formation of microtubules	Peripheral neuropathy
Cisplatin/ Carboplatin	Causes cross-linking of DNA	Hypomagnesaemia, ototoxicty, alopecia, peripheral neuropathy
Bleomycin	Degrades preformed DNA	Lung fibrosis
Docetaxel	Prevents microtubule disassembly	Neutropaenia
Doxorubicin	Inhibits RNA and DNA synthesis	Cardiomyopathy
Methotrexate	Inhibits dihydrofolate reductase	Myelosuppression, mucositis
Cyclophosphamide	Alkylating agent	Haemorrhagic cystitis, transitional cell carcinoma, myelosuppression
Fluorouracil (5-FU)	An anti-metabolite	Diarrhoea, mucositis, myelosuppression

Monoclonal antibody therapy and their application
Produced by Somatic cell hybridisation.

- Imatinib – tyrosine kinase inhibitor – treatment of CML.
- Infliximab – anti-TNF agent – used in Rheumatoid arthritis, IBD.
- Rituximab – anti-CD20 – used in treatment of NHL.
- Cetuximab – anti-epidermal growth factor – used in Colon carcinoma.
- Trastuzumab – anti-HER2 – used in HER2 positive breast cancer, is cardiotoxic.
- Alentuzumab – anti-CD52 – treatment of CLL.
- Abciximab – anti – glycoprotein IIb/IIIa – treatment of MI.

Tumour Lysis syndrome
- Due to sudden and large-scale cell death following initiation of chemotherapy.
- Seen in rapidly growing tumours, acute leukaemias and those that are most treatment sensitive. Can also identify those at high risk with a high serum LDH prior to treatment.

Features:
- hypocalcaemia
- acute renal failure
- hyperkalaemia
- elevated urate
- hyperphosphataemia.

Treatment – try to identify those at high risk. Ensure adequate IV hydration, urine alkalisation and prophylactic Allopurinol can be used.

Post cranial irradiation somnolence syndrome
Occurs following cranial radiotherapy. Two windows of occurrence, 11–21 days and 31–35 days post radiotherapy.

Features:
- excessive somnolence
- lethargy
- clumsiness.

It usually spontaneously resolves and requires no intervention.

Oncological associations
Erythropoietin secreting tumours (CURL)
Cerebellar haemangiomas.
Uterine fibromas.
Renal cell carcinoma.
Liver hepatoma.

All the above tumours may present with polycythaemia.

Thymoma associations
- Myasthenia gravis.
- Red cell aplasia.
- Dermatomyositis.
- SLE.
- SIADH.
- Pemphigoid vulgaris.

Haematinic deficiency
B$_{12}$ deficiency
- B$_{12}$ vital for erythropoiesis and maintenance of the nervous system.
- Binds to intrinsic factor, produced by gastric parietal cells, and is absorbed at the terminal ileum.

Causes of deficiency:
- poor diet
- pernicious anaemia

- gastrectomy
- terminal ileum disease, e.g. Crohn's
- Metformin.

Features:
- macrocytic anaemia
- glossitis
- ataxia
- confusion
- peripheral neuropathy – affects dorsal column, i.e. proprioception and vibration.

Treatment is replacement therapy. If there is co-existing folate deficiency it is essential to replace B_{12} first to prevent subacute degeneration of the cord.

Iron deficiency
Causes:
- blood loss – common in menstruating women, if seen in males > 55 years old should prompt investigation of GI tract
- poor diet
- malabsorption – Coeliac, Crohn's.

Features:
- microcytic anaemia
- koilonychia
- angular stomatitis
- atrophic glossitis
- post-cricoid web (Plummer Vision syndrome).

Investigations:
- blood film – target cells and 'pencil' poikilocytes
- low iron and ferritin levels, raised TIBC.

Chapter 9

Neurology

Neurological syndromes

Brown-Sequard syndrome

Is caused by lateral hemisection of the spinal cord.

Causes:

- trauma
- tumours
- MS.

Features:

- ipsilateral upper motor neurone (UMN) weakness (corticospinal tract)
- ipsilateral loss of proprioception and vibration sensation (dorsal column)
- contralateral loss of pain and temperature (crossed spinothalamic).

Lateral medullary syndrome (Wallenberg's syndrome)

Due to occlusion of either a vertebral artery or posterior inferior cerebellar artery (ipsilateral to resulting Horner's).

Features:

- ipsilateral Horner's
- ataxia
- CN V, VI, VII and VIII palsy.
- contralateral loss of pain and temperature sensation (spinothalamic).

Restless leg syndrome

Has an equal incidence between males and females.

Features:

- uncomfortable sensation in legs
- uncontrolled motor restlessness
- typically worse at night
- 50% have positive family history.

Associations:

- iron deficiency
- DM
- uraemia
- pregnancy.

Treatment – Ropinerole (dopamine agonist).

Normal pressure hydrocephalus

- Secondary to reduced CSF absorption at the arachnoid villi, therefore have accumulation of CSF and increased pressure.

Features (sudden change noticed by relatives/patient):

- dementia
- incontinence
- gait disturbance
- enlarged ventricle on imaging of the brain.

Treatment – ventriculoperitoneal shunt.

Bickerstaff's encephalitis

Most commonly follows a non-CNS viral illness.

Features:

- symmetrical opthalmoplegia
- ataxia

- reduced GCS
- up going plantars.

Treatment – steroids and IV Ig. Plasma exchange can be considered.

Weber's syndrome
Is a syndrome resulting from stroke, usually infarction of midbrain, features are:
- ipsilateral CN III palsy
- contralateral hemiplegia.

Hemiballismus
- Hemiballismus is usually characterised by involuntary flinging motions of the extremities, usually unilateral.
- Due to ipsilateral lesions within the subthalamic nucleus.

Causes:
- stroke
- trauma
- tumour
- AV malformations
- MS plaques.

Degenerative disease and neuropathy
Spinal tracts
With anterior spinal artery occlusion there is sparing of the dorsal column, therefore vibration, light touch and proprioception are preserved.

Polyneuropathy
Sensory neuropathy can occur in two manners.

1 Demyelinating:
- nerve conduction studies show reduced velocity, normal amplitude and absent F waves.

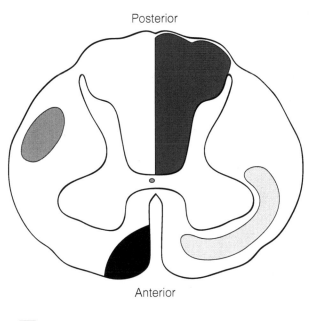

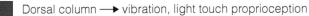

Figure 9.1 Spinal tracts

Causes:

- chronic inflammatory demyelinating polyneuropathy
- HIV
- Refsum's disease
- GBS
- amiodarone
- hereditary motor sensory neuropathy type 1.

2 Axonal:

- nerve conduction studies show reduced amplitude and normal velocity.

Causes:

- alcohol
- DM
- vasculitis
- renal failure
- B_{12} deficiency.

- Alcohol and DM are the most common causes of peripheral neuropathy.
- Vitamin B_{12} deficiency only affects the dorsal column, therefore see loss of proprioception and vibration.
- Lead neuropathy is purely motor, and mainly upper limbs.
- DM, uraemia, Vit B_{12}, alcohol and amyloidosis predominately result in sensory neuropathy.

Features of upper limb neuropathy

- Ulna nerve:
  - loss of thumb adduction
  - wasting of hypothenar eminence
  - weakness of flexion of little finger
  - loss of medial palmar sensation.

- Median nerve:
  - loss of lateral palmar sensation
  - wasting of thenar eminence
  - weakness of opposition and abduction of the thumb
  - weakness of lumbricals.

- Radial nerve:
  - wrist drop
  - loss of sensation on dorsum of hand.

Features of lower limb neuropathy

- Femoral nerve (L2–L4):
  - weakness of quadriceps

– sensation over anterior aspect of thigh
– reduced/absent knee reflex.

- Obturator nerve (L2–L4):
  – weakness of hip adductors
  – loss of sensation over lateral thigh.

- Common peroneal nerve (L4 root):
  – sensory loss over lateral aspect of calf and dorsum of foot
  – foot drop.

Cranial nerve palsies

- CN III (occulomotor):
  – ptosis
  – down and out gaze
  – pupil fixed and dilated (may be spared in vascular lesion).

Causes:

- posterior communicating artery aneurysm (painful)
- DM
- cavernous sinus pathology
- tumour
- trauma
- herniation.

- CN IV (trochlear):
  – loss of downward gaze
  – vertical diplopia.

Causes:

- vascular
- DM
- congenital
- trauma
- cavernous sinus pathology.

- CN VI:
  - innervates lateral rectus
  - loss of lateral gaze
  - medial deviation of eye, due to unopposed action of medial rectus.

Causes:
- SOL
- vascular
- MS
- cavernous sinus pathology
- migraine.

- CN VII:
  - innervates the muscles of the face
  - there is bilateral innervation of frontalis, therefore in UMN lesions there is sparing of frontalis whilst in LMN there is not.

Causes:
- LMN
- Bell's palsy
- Ramsay Hunt syndrome
- MS
- GBS
- Lyme disease
- UMN
- stroke
- tumour
- MS
- syphilis.

- CN VIII:
  - results in sensorineural deafness and vertigo
  - can use Webber's and Rinne's testing to distinguish type of deafness.

Causes of sensorineural deafness:

- acoustic neuromas
- Paget's disease
- congenital
- trauma
- drugs – Gentamicin, Furosemide.

Motor neurone disease

- Is a degenerative condition of the anterior horn cells. As a result it affects UMN and LMN supply of lower limb, upper limb and bulbar muscles. There is no involvement of sensory nerves.
- Three main types.

1 Progressive muscular atrophy:
- presents with LMN signs affecting a single limb and then progresses to affect others.

2 Amyotrophic lateral sclerosis:
- is the most common clinical pattern
- LMN signs in the arms, with bilateral LMN signs in the legs.

3 Progressive bulbar palsy:
- progressive involvement of bulbar muscles, carries the worst prognosis.

Features:
- fasciculations
- wasting
- weakness
- spastic dysarthria
- hyperreflexia.

Diagnosis is mainly clinically, but NCS and EMG studies can be used to confirm.

·Prognosis is poor with limited treatment options.

Guillain–Barré syndrome (GBS)

- Is an immune mediated demyelinating process, resulting in polyneuropathy.
- Commonly follows a viral infection, can be seen following *Campylobacter jejuni* infection, this carries a poor prognosis.

Features:
- ascending symmetrical muscle weakness
- areflexia
- loss of plantar response
- autonomic involvement, e.g. urinary retention, postural hypotension.

Investigations:
- elevated protein levels of CSF analysis
- slow nerve conduction
- anti-GM1 antibody positive.

Treatment:
- IV immunoglobulin
- it is essential to establish baseline FVC and use this to assess ascendance of neuropathy. If falling patient will require ventilatory support.

Poor prognosis:
- > 40 years old
- associated with *Campylobacter*
- high Anti-GM1 antibody levels
- poor upper body muscle strength prior.

Miller Fisher

- Is a variant of GBS.
- See opthalmoplegia, ataxia, areflexia and affects the upper limbs first.

- Descending paralysis.
- Anti-GQ1b antibody positive.

Causes:
- Hep B
- EBV
- CMV
- herpes zoster
- *mycoplasma* pneumonia.

Creutzfeldt–Jakob disease
- A prion disease.

Characterised by:
- young age at onset
- rapidly progressive dementia
- myoclonus
- biphasic EEG changes.

Two types.

1 Sporadic CJD – associated with characteristic biphasic, high amplitude sharp waves on EEG and FLAIR MRI series.
2 New variant CJD – due to Bovine Spongiform Encephalopathy (BSE). Diagnosed via characteristic changes in posterior thalamus on MRI.

No treatment available.

Myasthenia Gravis
- An autoimmune disorder.
- Autoantibodies produced that block the acetylcholine receptors of the post-synaptic neuromucular junction. As a result they reduced neuronal stimulation of muscles.
- More common in females.

Features:
- ptosis
- extra-occular muscle weakness
- fatiguability
- proximal muscle weakness
- dysphagia.

Associated with thymomas and other autoimmune disease, e.g. SLE, hypothyroidism. Relapse may be seen during pregnancy.

Investigation:
- positive antibody testing, both acetylcholine receptor and MuSK
- tensilon test positive
- NCS and EMG.

Exacerbating drugs:
- Penicillamine
- Beta Blockers
- Lithium
- Gentamicin
- Quinidine
- Ciprofloxacin
- Phenytoin.

Treatment:
- long acting acetylcholinesterase inhibitors – Pyridostigmine
- steroids
- thymectomy
- in MG crisis Plasmapheresis and/or IV Ig can be used.

Visual field defects and pupil disorder
Optic pathway and visual field defects
See Figure 9.2 opposite.

1   Central scotoma – optic neuritis

2   Occular blindness – transection of optic nerve

3   Bitemporal hemianopia – optic chiasm compression

4   Superior quadrantanopia – temporal lobe lesion

5   Inferior quadrantanopia – parietal lobe lesion

6   Homonymous hemianopia – occipital lesion

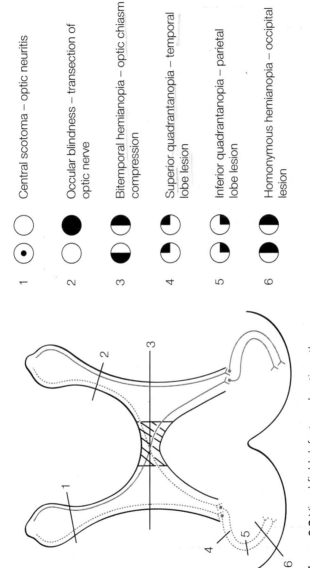

Figure 9.2 Visual field defects and optic pathway

Pupil disorder

Small pupil (miosis):

- senile pupil
- pontine haemorrhage
- Horner's syndrome
- Argyll Robertson pupil
- drugs – opiates, Pilocarpine
- myotonic dystrophy
- DM.

Large pupil (mydriasis):

- Holmes-Adie's pupil
- CNIII palsy
- drugs – atropine, cobalt, ethylene glycol, TCA, amphetamines
- sphincter pupillae rupture
- herniation.

Stroke and venous thrombosis

Stroke classification

Total Anterior Circulation Stroke (TACS):

- higher cerebral function, ipsilateral sensory/motor defect and visual field affected.

Partial Anterior Circulation Stroke (PACS):

- two of the above or new higher cerebral function disorder.

Lacunar Circulation Stroke (LACS):

- pure motor or sensory, or ataxia, or dysarthria.

Posterior Circulation Stroke (POCS):

- bilateral motor/sensory loss, visual field defect, CN or cerebellar dysfunction.

Lobar strokes

Strokes affecting specific lobes of the brain will have distinctive presentations.

Occipital:
- contralateral homonymous heminopia
- cortical blindness
- visual agnosia.

Frontal:
- expressive aphasia/dysphasia
- preservation
- primitive reflexes affected
- anosmia
- urinary and faecal incontinence.

Parietal:
- inferior homonymous quadrantonopia
- apraxias
- visuospacial neglect
- acalculia
- astereognosis.

Temporal:
- superior homonymous quadrantonopia
- receptive aphasia
- memory impairment
- auditory agnosia.

Cerebral autosomal dominant arteriopathy with subcortical infarcts and leukoencephalopathy (CADASIL)

- Is a rare, genetic cause for stroke, autosomal dominant, therefore has positive family history, usually at a young age.
- A disease of small arteries.

Features:

- history of migraine with aura
- recurrent ischaemic events (TIA or stroke)
- mood disorder
- sub-cortical dementia
- leukoencephalopathy on MRI
- thalamus and basal ganglia frequently affected.

CT is non-diagnostic, requires MRI and NOTCH-3 genetic testing.

Venous sinus thrombosis

Describes thrombosis within the dural venous sinuses.

Causes:

- OCP
- pregnancy and post-partum period
- hypercoaguable states, e.g. malignancy, nephrotic syndrome, Behçet's, SLE.

Features:

- symptoms of stroke
- headache
- seizure
- papilloedema
- CN III, IV and VI palsy – ocular chemosis, also see proptosis.

Diagnosis via CT/MRI venogram.

Treatment – anticoagulation, initially heparin and then Warfarin.

Cavernous sinus disease

Structures that pass through the cavernous sinus are:

- CN III, IV, V_1 and VI
- internal carotid artery.

Lesions in this region may therefore cause total internal or external opthalmoplegia.

Causes:
- trauma
- vascular – aneurysm
- sinus thrombosis
- tumour
- Wegener's.

Headache

Chronic recurrent headache can be classified as:
- tension
- migraine
- cluster
- benign intracranial hypertension.

Tension
- Arises from tension within the muscles of the head and neck.
- Typically frontal and generalised.
- Occur towards the end of the day.
- Usually respond to analgesics.
- Must ensure headache not due to chronic analgesic use.

Migraine
- Due to vascular spasm around the head.
- Described as a unilateral throbbing headache, associated with photophobia and nausea.
- It may be preceded by aura, e.g. scotoma, fortification spectra.

Other features:
- CN III palsy
- hemiplegia

- delayed gastric emptying
- increased risk of stroke.

Triggers:
- chocolate
- alcohol
- pregnancy
- meat
- citrus fruit.

Treatment:
- abortive:
  - 5HT1 agonists Sumatriptan
  - paracetamol
  - codeine.
- Prophylactic:
  - propanolol
  - TCA
  - Pizotifen.

Cluster

- Most commonly seen in males.
- Usually nocturnal.

Features:
- head described as peri-orbital and unilateral
- lacrimation
- ptosis
- pupil constriction
- nasal congestion
- red eye.

Treatment:
- acute – SC Sumatriptan and high flow oxygen
- prophylactic – Verapamil, Prednisalone or Lithium.

Benign intracranial hypertension

Affects overweight young females.

Features:
- headache
- papilloedema
- normal CSF analysis
- normal imaging of the brain
- horizontal diplopia
- enlarged blind spot.

Causes:
- obesity
- drugs – steroids, tetracyclines, Vit A, Nitrofurantoin
- OCP.

Treatment:
- weight loss
- Acetazolamide
- repeated LP and CSF removal
- V-P shunt.

Diagnostic neurological auto-antibodies

- Anti-muscle specific kinase antibody – Myasthenia Gravis.
- Anti GQib antibody – Miller Fisher syndrome.
- Anti voltage gated calcium channel antibody – Lambert-Eaton syndrome.
- Anti GM1 antibody – ALS, MS, GBS, SLE with neuro involvement.
- HU antibody – small cell paraneoplastic syndrome.
- Anti-Yo antibody – cerebellar syndrome associated with ovarian and breast.
- Purkinje cell antibody –peripheral neuropathy in breast cancer.

- Anti-Ri antibody – ocular opsoclonus-myoclonus, breast and small cell lung cancer.

Herpes simplex encephalitis

- HSV-1 responsible for 95% of cases.
- Most commonly affects the temporal lobe.

Features:
- fever
- headache
- seizures
- aphasia/dysphasia
- cold sores have no relation to encephalitis.

Investigation:
- LP – lymphocytosis, elevated protein, positive PCR for HSV
- CT – petechial haemorrhage, commonly frontal and temporal lobes
- MRI – enhancement of temporal lobes
- EEG –lateralised periodic 2Hz discharges.

Treatment – should not be delayed, if suspected to commence IV Aciclovir.

Movement disorder
Chorea
Arises from damage to the caudate nucleus.

Causes:
- Huntington's disease
- SLE
- Wilson's disease, Sydenham's chorea – following rheumatic fever

- Drugs – Levodopa, OCP, CO poisoning
- chorea gravidarum
- thyrotoxicosis.

Huntington's disease:
- a CAG trinucleotide repeat disorder
- autosomal dominant
- defect seen on chromosome 4
- shows anticipation
- along with the chorea there is cognitive decline, dysarthria, dysphagia, ataxia and myoclonus.

Parkinsonism
Refers to a triad of:
- resting tremor
- bradykinesia
- rigidity (cogwheel).

Causes:
- idiopathic Parkinson's disease
- drug induced
- toxins – manganese, MPTP
- Wilson's disease
- normal pressure hydrocephalus
- Lewy body disease
- dementia pugilistica
- CJD
- progressive supranuclear palsy
- corticobasal degeneration
- multiple system atrophy.

Distinguishing features of idiopathic Parkinson's disease are:
- asymmetrical onset of symptoms
- persistent asymmetry
- good response to L-dopa.

Treatment of Parkinson's disease:
- is only started once symptoms become troublesome
- anticholinergics are used when tremor predominate, e.g. Benzhexol, Procyclidine
- L-dopa and dopamine agonist are useful for akinesia and bradykinesia.

Dopamine agonist – Cabergoline, Ropinerole, Apomorphine – may result in pulmonary, cardiac and retroperitoneal fibrosis.

Levodopa – combined with a decarboxylase inhibitor to reduce peripheral side effects – side effects are dyskinesia and on/off effect. MAO-B inhibitors – Selegiline, inhibit breakdown of dopamine.

Neurofibromatosis

There are two types.

- Type 1 (NF1, von Reckinghausen's disease):
  - chromosome 17, autosomal dominant
  - features are neurocutaneous.

Diagnosis is made if two of the following features are present:
- > 5 café-au-lait spots
- > 1 neurofibroma
- freckling in the axillary or inguinal region
- optic glioma
- > 1 lisch nodule on iris
- first-degree relative with NF1 according to above criteria.

Complications of NF1:
- nerve root compression
- spinal cord compression
- renal artery stenosis
- phaeochromocytoma
- optic glioma.

- Type 2 (NF2):
  - chromosome 22, autosomal dominant
  - associated with bilateral acoustic neuromas.

Diagnosis is made if either of the following is found:
- bilateral vestibular schwannomas
- first-degree relative with NF2 and either:
  - unilateral vestibular schwannoma
  - neurofibroma
  - meningioma
  - glioma
  - schwannoma.

Complications:
- malignant change
- deafness
- spinal cord/nerve root compression.

Tuberous sclerosis

- Autosomal dominant neurocutaneous disorder.
- Genes located on chromosomes 9 and 16.

Features:
- Ash-leaf spots
- Shagreen patches – esp over lumbosacral areas
- Adenoma sebaceum
- café-au-lait spots
- retinal hamartomas
- renal angiomyolipomata
- seizures
- infantile spasm
- delayed development and cognitive impairment.

Chapter 10
Rheumatology

Wegener's granulomatosis

- A systemic small/medium vasculitis with necrotising granulomatous inflammation. Commonly affects lungs, kidneys, nasal passages and skin.

Features:
- bloody nasal discharge
- crusting of nasal passages
- collapse of nasal bridge, leaving saddle shaped nose
- pulmonary haemorrhage
- multiple pulmonary nodules
- focal segmental glomerulonephritis, with renal failure
- vasculitic rash.

Investigations:
- CXR – pulmonary nodules, haemorrhage
- Bloods – ARF, cANCA positive, elevated ESR, thrombocytosis
- End organ damage is an indication for IV therapy.

Treatment:
- IV Methylprednisalone and Cyclophosphamide
- during initial treatment can consider PCP prophylaxis.

Takayasu's disease

- A granulomatous inflammatory process affecting the aorta and it branches.
- Most commonly affects females.

Features:
- fever, malaise and weight loss
- TIA
- claudication
- angina
- aortic regurgitation
- glomerulonephritis.

Treatment – steroids and DMARDs.

Goodpasture's disease

- Presents with a bimodal presentation.
- Young men typically with a pulmonary-renal picture, whilst elderly women present with renal involvement alone.
- Due to autoantibodies directs towards the Glomerular Basement Membrane (GBM).

Features:
- ARF, secondary to rapidly progressive GN
- pulmonary haemorrhage.

Investigations:
- ANCA positive
- anti-GBM antibody positive
- increased gas transfer due to pulmonary haemorrhage
- renal biopsy – IgG linear deposits along GBM and complement deposition.

Treatment:
- pulsed Methylprednisalone and Cyclophosphamide
- if have severe pulmonary haemorrhage can consider plasmapharesis to remove anti-GBM antibodies.

Dermatomyositis and polymyositis

- Polymyositis describes inflammation of the skeletal muscle, when it is associated with cutaneous changes it is termed Dermatomyositis.
- Is associated with an underlying malignancy, thus upon initial presentation should prompt further investigation.

Features:
- proximal muscles weakness and tenderness
- heliotrope purple rash around eyes and cheeks
- Gottron's papules on hands
- dilated capillary loops at nail folds
- fever
- arthritis
- myocarditis
- Raynaud's.

Investigations:
- elevated CK, AST and LDH
- abnormal EMG
- ANA and Anti-Jo-1 positive antibody testing.

Treatment:
- must extensively exclude malignancy
- immunosuppression, with steroids and steroid sparing agents.

Arthritides
Reactive arthritis
Consists of a triad of:
- uveitis
- arthritis
- urethritis.

Others – keratoderma blenorrhagica, pericarditis.

Results from infection elsewhere within the body:

- GUM – gonorrhoea, chlamydia
- GIT – *Shigella, campylobacter, salmonella*.

Investigation should look to culture for the above infections.

Treatment:

- treat underlying infection
- NSAIDS for arthritis
- can consider immune-modulation
- up to 50% will have recurrence of arthritis.

Psoriatic arthritis

- Represents a seronegative arthritis.
- Male and females are equally affected.
- It may precede the skin manifestation of psoriasis.

Five distinct patterns:

- asymmetrical oligoarthritis
- axial involvement
- rheumatoid arthritis like picture
- DIP involvement predominant
- arthritis mutilans (telescoping of fingers).

Other features:

- Nails – pitting and transverse ridging
- dactylitis
- enthesitis.

Treatment is with NSAIDs and immunosuppression.

Felty's syndrome

- Seen in seropositive rheumatoid arthritis, most common in females.
- ANA positive in 90%.

Features:
- leucopaenia
- splenomegaly
- lymphadenopathy
- flare of rheumatoid arthritis
- recurrent infection.

Treatment:
- DMARDs, particularly gold, with pulsed steroids
- splenectomy can be considered.

Key features of rheumatoid arthritis

Poor prognostic factors:
- positive rheumatoid factor
- extra-articular features
- HLA-DR4
- female sex
- early erosion
- insidious onset
- severe disability at presentation.

Extra-articular manifestations:
- rheumatoid nodules – most commonly at extensor surfaces, associated with more severe arthritis. May see pulmonary nodulation
- eye involvement – with scleritis and episcleritis
- vasculitis – varying severity in manifestation. From nail fold infarcts to mononeuritis multiplex and cerebral artery involvement
- cardio-respiratory – pericarditis, fibrosis, obliterative bronchiolitis, Caplan's syndrome
- Felty's syndrome
- anaemia
- amyloidosis
- pyoderma gangrenosum.

X-ray changes (early to late):
- soft tissue swelling
- joint space narrowing
- bone and joint destruction
- subluxation.

Infliximab therapy:
- is licensed for the treatment of active rheumatoid arthritis in combination with methotrexate when the response to other DMARDs is inadequate
- prior to each infusion important to measure FBC, UE and LFTs
- must rule out TB before commencing therapy.

Side effects:
- myelosuppression
- demyelination
- hepatitis
- cardiomyopathy.

Still's disease

Most commonly seen in children < 5 years of age. Can present in adulthood as adult onset Still's disease.

Features:
- swinging fever
- salmon pink rash
- serositis – large and small joints
- autoimmune screen normal
- generalised lymphadenopathy
- raised serum ferritin.

May progress to a destructive arthropathy.

Treatment is with NSAIDs.

Auto-antibody associations

SLE

- ANA – positive in up to 95%.
- Anti – dsDNA – very specific, used to measure disease activity.
- Anti-Sm – not common but when seen highly specific.

Dermatomyositis

- Anti-Jo-1.
- ANA.

Systemic sclerosis

- Anticentromere – up to 90% in CREST.
- Anti Scl 70.
- ANA.
- Rheumatoid factor.

Sjögrens

- ANA.
- Anti-Ro and Anti-La.
- Rheumatoid factor.

Congenital complete heart block and SLE

- Anti-Ro, anti-dsDNA may be present, but is not as specifically associated with CHB as anti-Ro.

Crystal arthropathy

Gout

Here hyperuricaemia leads to deposition of sodium monourate crystals in and around joints.

Causes:

- idiopathic
- increased uric acid production/intake – myeloproliferative disease, high purine diet (beer, red meat), acidosis, surgery

- decreased uric acid excretion – renal failure, drugs (diuretics, aspirin, Ciclosporin), alcohol.

Features:
- acute crystal arthritis – typically 1st MTP joint
- gout tophi – seen around hands and ears
- negatively birefringent crystals on aspiration of joints.

Treatment:
- acute – NSAIDs and/or Colchicine (side effect of diarrhoea is common)
- prophylaxis-lifestyle changes, drug avoidance:
  - Allopurinol (not to be started during acute attacks).

Calcium pyrophosphate dihydrate (CPPD) arthropathy

When occurs as an acute monoarthritis is termed pseudogout.

Risk factors:
- dehydration
- hyperparathyroidism
- low serum phosphate and magnesium
- haemochromatosis
- acromegaly.

Similar presentation to gout, distinguished by the presence of positively birefringent crystals. See chondrocalcinosis on X-ray of joints.

Treatment:
- steroid can be used in the acute phase
- consider Hydroxychloroquine for chronic disease.

Paget's disease

- Disorder of osteoclast and osteoblast activity, as a result see excessive lysis and sclerosis.
- More common in females.

Features:
- bone pain
- bone deformity
- CN II, V, VII and VIII compression
- high output cardiac failure
- pathological fracture
- increased risk of bone sarcoma (rare).

Blood – high Alk phos, normal Calcium and Phosphate.

Typically changes seen on X-rays.

Treatment – Bisphosphanates.

Behçet's disease

An immune mediated occlusive vasculitis and venulitis, with a multi-organ presentation.

Features:
- oral ulceration
- genital ulceration
- irisitis
- thrombosis
- erythaema nodosum.

Seen in those from the Middle East and eastern Mediterranean.

Drug induced Lupus

- Able to distinguish between non-drug induced Lupus as antihistone antibodies are positive and Complement 3 and 4 are normal (reduced in SLE).
- Male and female predominance equal.

Causes:

- Hydralazine
- Minocycline
- Quinine
- Captopril
- Sulfazalasine
- Simvastatin
- Phenytoin
- Isoniazid.

Baker's cyst associations

- TB.
- Gout.
- SLE.
- Hypothyroidism.
- Psoriasis.
- Sarcoidosis.
- Dialysis.

Chapter 11

Endocrine and diabetes

Thyroid dysfunction

Hyperthyroidism

Causes:

- Graves' disease
- toxic multinodular goitre
- toxic nodule
- thyroiditis
- ectopic thyroid tissue.

Symptoms and signs (divided by system affected):

- GI – diarrhoea, weight loss
- CVS – AF, high output cardiac failure
- musculoskeletal – proximal myopathy, osteoporosis, hypercalcaemia, tremor
- Gynae – amenorrhoea, raised sex hormone binding globulin
- blood – leucopaenia, microcytic anaemia.

Hypothyroidism

Causes:

- spontaneous primary atrophic
- post-thyroidectomy or radioiodine treatment
- drug induced
- iodine deficiency
- subacute thyroiditis.

Symptoms and signs (divided by system affected):

- GI-constipation, weight gain
- CVS-IHD, hypercholesterolaemia
- musculoskeletal – myalgia, elevated CK, cramps
- Gynae – menorrhagia, infertility
- skin – dry skin, periorbital oedema
- blood – macrocytic anaemia.

Graves' disease

- TSH receptors are subject to auto-antibody stimulation.
- There is diffuse enlargement of the thyroid gland.
- Uniform uptake with technetium scanning.

Auto-antibodies:

- anti-TSH receptor stimulating antibody (90%)
- anti-thyroid peroxidase antibody (50%).

See specific Graves' related eye disease:

- proptosis/exopthalmus
- diplopia/opthalmoplegia
- optic nerve compression.

Association:

- elevated ESR
- hypercalcaemia
- Type 1 DM
- pernicious anaemia
- deranged LFTs.

Orbital radiotherapy can be used to reduced eye disease. Those with eye disease who have radioiodine therapy may initially have worsening symptoms.

DeQuervains thyroiditis (subacute thyroiditis)
Commonly follows a viral infection or URTI.

Features:

- self limiting
- painful enlargement, with fever
- initially hyperthyroid, becoming hypothyroid
- reduced TSH
- reduced ^{123}I uptake on isotope scan.

Treatment – NSAIDs +/– Prednisalone.

Thyroid storm

- Seen in patients who are previously thyrotoxic.
- Not due to excess thyroxine treatment.

Feature:

- fever
- tachycardia
- hypertension
- agitation
- abnormal LFTs
- nausea
- vomiting.

Treatment:

- Propanolol
- Lugols iodine
- Methinazole or Propylthiouracil
- Dexamethasone, can be used to block conversion of T_4 to T_3.

Subclinical hyperthyroidism

Defined when:

- normal T_4 and T_3
- TSH below normal.

Caused by multinodular goitre and may be seen with excessive thyroxine. Patients have the potential to develop AF/SVT and osteoporosis, therefore warrants treatment.

Treatment:
- can resolve spontaneously, however treatment with low dose Carbimazole used. Acts via the inhibition of iodination of tyrosine.

Subclinical hypothyroidism
Defined when:
- TSH raised
- normal T_4 and T_3
- no signs of disease.

There is a risk of progressing to overt hypothyroidism, this risk is increased by the presence of thyroid antibody.

Treat with replacement therapy if:
- TSH >10 mmol/l
- thyroid antibody positive
- previous Graves' disease
- other autoimmune disease.

Gestational thyrotoxicosis
- During pregnancy there is a rise in thyroxin-binding globulin, therefore have increase in total thyroxine.
- Graves' disease is the most common cause of Thyrotoxicosis during pregnancy.
- Beta-HCG can also stimulate TSH receptors.

Complications:
- fetal loss
- premature labour
- maternal heart failure.

Treatment – Propylthiouracil.

Amiodarone induced thyroid disease
Can result in both hypo and hyperthyroidism.

Hyperthyroidism caused in two ways.

Type 1 – due to excess iodine found in Amiodarone.
Type 2 – acute thyroiditis, see reduced uptake on isotope scanning.

Treatment:
- stop Amiodarone, however may persist for months afterwards
- Carbimazole can be used and Prednisalone added in Type 2.

Thyroid cancer
May not have any thyroid dysfunction.

- Papillary – 70%, often young females, good prognosis.
- Follicular – 20%.
- Medullary – 5%, seen as part of MEN II, secrete Calcitonin.
- Anaplastic – 1%, poor response to treatment.
- Lymphoma – associated with prior Hashimoto's thyroiditis.

Papillary thyroid carcinoma:
- slow growing and may spread to cervical lymph nodes
- thyroglobulin used as a marker of recurrence after resection.

Risks – excessive iodine, external radiation to the neck.

Associated with FAP, Gardener's and Cowden disease.

Radioactive ^{131}I treatment
- Seventy per cent of those treated have hypothyroidism after three months.
- No risk of infertility or lymphoma.
- Can initially make Graves' worse.
- Cannot be used in Amiodarone induced thyroid disease.

Adrenal dysfunction

Cushing's

- Syndrome – elevated levels of cortisol.
- Disease – secondary to elevated levels of ACTH.

Causes:

- ACTH dependent:
  - pituitary tumour (80%)
  - ectopic site e.g. small cell lung cancer.
- ACTH independent:
  - steroids
  - adenoma of the adrenal gland.

Features:

- symptoms:
  - weight gain
  - amenorrhoea
  - reduced libido
  - acne.
- signs:
  - necrosis of femoral head
  - moon face
  - abdominal striae
  - osteoporosis and fractures
  - proximal myopathy
  - hypertension
  - hirsuitism
  - hypokalaemia and metabolic alkalosis.

Investigation:

- 24 or 48 hour Dexamethasone suppression test and ACTH level
- the ACTH can be used to defined 'disease' and localise, i.e. pituitary or ectopic site
- if ACTH is raised then MRI of brain is indicated.

Addison's disease

- Represents adrenal insufficiency.
- Eighty per cent due to autoimmune destruction by Anti-21 hydroxylase antibodies, commonly seen with other autoimmune conditions and in women.

Other causes:

- HIV
- TB
- adrenal mets
- post meningococcal septicaemia (Waterhouse-Friderichsen syndrome).

Features:

- hyponatraemia
- hypoglycaemia
- hypotension
- pyrexia
- increased skin pigmentation
- abdominal pain
- nausea and vomiting
- reduced dihydroepiandrosterone, leading to reduced libido.

Can present an acute crisis with severe hypotension, hypoglycaemia and hyponatraemia.

Treatment – steroid replacement therapy, hydrocortisone.

Hyperaldosteronism

Can be divided into primary and secondary.

- Primary – excess production of aldosterone independent of the renin-angiotensin system. Should be considered if have hypokalaemia, hypertension and alkalosis, in a patient not on diuretics. The most common primary cause is Conn's syndrome, caused by a unilateral active adenoma.

- Secondary – excess levels of renin, e.g. renal artery stenosis, CCF, hepatic failure.

Investigation:
- uses postural changes in cortisol, aldosterone and renin
- low cortisol and aldosterone on standing – Conn's
- low cortisol and raised aldosterone on standing – angiotensin II dependent.

Treatment:
- in Conn's surgical removal of the adenoma is required
- Spironolactone is an effective treatment for other causes.

Congenital adrenal hyperplasia

Due to a group of recessively inherited enzyme deficiency disorder. There are two principle effects seen:

1   low cortisol +/– low aldosterone
2   excess precursor steroids.

In response there is elevated ACTH from the pituitary and hyperplasia of the adrenal gland.

Features:
- clitoral hypertrophy and fusion of the labia
- amenorrhoea
- infertility
- precocious puberty
- addisonian crisis in first weeks of life, may result in death
- premature epiphyseal closure
- hyponatraemia
- hypoglycaemia.

Treatment – hydrocortisone and salt retaining fludrocortisone.

Hypertension and hypokalaemia

To distinguish the causes of hypokalaemia the presence of hypertension can be used.

Hypokalaemia + hypertension:
- Cushing's
- Conn's
- Liddle's
- 11 Beta hydroxylase deficiency.

Hypokalaemia + normotensive:
- diuretics
- GI loss
- renal tubular acidosis
- Bartter's syndrome
- Gitelman's syndrome.

Phaeochromocytoma

A rare catecholamine producing tumour, arise from the adrenal medullar, with 90% being unilateral.

Associations:
- MEN2a
- neurofibromatosis
- von Hippel-Lindau syndrome.

Features – are typically episodic and can last minute to days:
- chest tightness
- sweating
- tachycardia and palpitations
- tremor
- flushing
- dyspnoea
- syncope
- abdominal pain.

There will also be hypertension and glycosuria during attacks.

Investigation – 24 hour catecholamine collection and imaging of adrenals CT/MRI.

Treatment:
- hypertension control is required before any surgery; this is achieved with alpha blocker phenoxybenzamine being given before a cardioselective beta blocker
- surgical removal of the tumour is curative.

Pituitary dysfunction

Acromegaly
- Due to excessive production of growth hormone (GH) from the pituitary gland.
- Results from Gs protein alpha subunit mutation.
- Typically presenting between the ages of 30 and 50 years.

Features:
- those of intracranial SOL
- bitemporal heminopia due to optic chiasm compression
- excessive soft tissue growth
  - large hands and feet
  - large tongue
  - increased spacing of the teeth
  - prominent supraorbital ridge
  - deepening of the voice.
- insulin resistance.

Complications:
- hypertension
- DM
- cardiomyopathy
- colorectal cancer

- pseudogout
- hyperthyroidism with goitre
- hyperphosphataemia.

Investigation:
- oral glucose tolerance test – failure to suppress serum GH levels
- this should be followed by pituitary fossa imaging, i.e. MRI
- test the rest of pituitary hormone with dynamic testing.

Treatment:
- surgery is the form of Trans-sphenoidal resection is first line
- medical therapies – Somatostatin analogues (Octreotide), Pegvisomant (GH receptor antagonist, does not reduce tumour volume).

Diabetes insipidus and water deprivation testing
- Due to reduced activity of AHD, either due to reduced secretion from posterior pituitary (cranial), or impaired response of the collecting systems of the nephrons (nephrogenic).

Symptoms are polyuria, thirst, polydipsia, severe dehydration if not drinking enough.

Causes:
- cranial:
  - head injury
  - pituitary surgery
  - sarcoidosis
  - histocytosis
  - pituitary metastases.
- nephrogenic:
  - lithium
  - hypercalcaemia

- sickle cell anaemia
- hypokalaemia
- Demeclocycline.

Investigation:
- plasma osmolality should be raised and urine reduced
- serum sodium can be raised
- to define the cause a water deprivation test can be used.

Table 11.1 Water deprivation test findings

	Starting plasma osmolality mmoL/kg	Final urine osmolality mmoL/kg	Urine osmolality mmoL/kg
Normal	Normal	< 600	> 600
Psychogenic	Low	> 400	> 400
Cranial	High	< 300	> 600
Nephrogenic	High	< 300	< 300

Treatment:
- cranial – isolate and correct any cause, then Desmopressin
- nephrogenic – remove underlying cause.

Hyperprolactinaemia
- Prolactin is released from the anterior pituitary; this release is inhibited by dopamine. Therefore hyperprolactinaemia can arise in two ways. Either by excess anterior pituitary secretion or failed inhibition by dopamine. The latter occurring with compression of the pituitary stalk or antagonistic drugs.

Causes:
- Prolactinoma
- pituitary adenoma
- stalk compression
- CRF
- Haloperidol

- Metoclopramide
- Methyldopa
- sarcoidosis.

Features:
- weight gain
- reduced libido
- apathy
- galactorrhoea
- amenorrhoea
- symptoms and sign of cranial SOL
- impotence.

Treatment:
- trans-sphenoidal surgery is used to remove prolactinomas, pituitary ademonas and can be used to decompress the stalk
- dopamine agonist are the medical option, used in an adjuvant role, e.g. Bromocriptine, Carbogoline.

Autoimmune polyendocrinopathy syndrome
Two types.

- Type 1 – chronic mucocutaneous candidiasis, Addison's disease, hypoparathyroidism.
- Type 2 – Addison's disease, hypothyroidism, DM type 1, hypogonadism, coeliac, myasthenia gravis.

Diabetes mellitus (DM)

Diagnosis of DM
If suspect DM, then fasting blood glucose required for diagnosis. A high random blood glucose is not diagnostic.

Fasting glucose results:
- < 6.1 mmol/l – normal

- 6.1–6.9 mmol/l – impaired fasting glycaemia, this will require further investigation with Oral Glucose Tolerance Test (OGTT)
- > 6.9 mmol/l diagnostic of DM.

Oral Glucose Tolerance Test (OGTT):
- < 7.8 – normal
- 2 hour value > 11.1 diagnostic of DM
- 7.8–11 – impaired glucose tolerance testing.

Twenty-five per cent of people when first diagnosed with DM have presented with DKA.

Genetic association
Type 1:
- autoimmune Beta cell destruction
- 40% concordance between twins
- associated with HLA DR3 and DR4
- polygenic inheritance.

Type 2:
- relative insulin resistance and deficiency
- 90% concordance between twins
- no HLA association.

Maturity onset diabetes of the young (MODY)
- See development of Type 2 DM in patients under 25 years of age.
- Autosomal dominant, therefore will have positive family history.
- Due to defect on *HNF 1 alpha* gene, resulting in glucokinase mutation.

Treatment of DM[5]
- Target HbA1C is 6.5%.
- BP target is < 140/80 or < 130/80 if have end organ damage, ACE-inhibitors first line.

- Lifestyle advice is first treatment option, unless there is end organ damage.

Metformin:
- act to increase insulin sensitivity, reduces hepatic gluconeogenesis and increase muscle utilisation. Requires some islet cell production of insulin
- first line in obese diabetic patients
- risk of lactic acidosis in hepatic and renal failure, if creatinine > 150 mmol/l should be stopped
- stop for 6 weeks following MI, and for 48 hours post IV contrast
- side effect of diarrhoea and B12 deficiency with macrocytic anaemia.

Glitazones (Thiazolidinediones):
- PPAR-gamma receptor agonist, reduces peripheral insulin resistance
- second line therapy
- aim for > 0.5% reduction in HbA1C after 6 months of treatment.
- avoid in heart failure.

Side effects:
- Weight gain
- Fluid retention
- Hepatic impairment
- Increase in fractures.

Sulphonylureas:
- augment insulin secretion, therefore can only be active if there is residual beta cell function
- is considered in those who are not overweight, or in whom Metformin is not tolerated
- there is a risk of hypoglycaemia, if it does occur it can persist for several hours

- cP450 interaction
- GI disturbance is the main side effect.

Exenatide:
- mimics the effects of Glucagon-like Peptide 1 (GLP-1)
- results in increased insulin release, suppressed appetite, delayed gastric emptying and reduced hepatic gluconeogenesis
- causes weight loss
- GI disturbance, namely nausea and vomiting, are the main side effects.

Diagnosis of metabolic syndrome
Require three of:
- central obesity
- Triglycerides > 1.7 mmol/l
- HDL < 1.03 mmol/l
- hypertension > 130/85
- DM.

Insulinoma

- A tumour derived from Islet of Langerhan cells.
- Can be part of MEN I.

Features:
- recurrent hypoglycaemic attacks – typically in the morning
- rapid weight gain
- elevated C-peptide.

- A supervised prolonged fast is used for diagnosis. When the patient becomes hypoglycaemic, serum insulin and C-peptide levels are taken. They will be abnormally high. CT pancreas is used to image.
- When insulin is released normally C peptide is also released, therefore with endogenous insulin see raised levels.

- If there is excess exogenous insulin there is reduced C peptide, e.g. in insulin abuse.

Carcinoid syndrome

- Neuroendocrine tumour that secretes serotonin.
- Arise from the GI tract and/or lungs.
- See Carcinoid syndrome when Vasoactive substances enter the systemic circulation and avoid hepatic degradation.
- The left side of the heart is usually unaffected as the lung clear serotonin. A lung tumour is required to produce left sided heart disease.

Features:
- flushing
- diarrhoea
- hypotension
- bronchospasm
- right heart valve disease
- Pellagra.

Investigation:
- elevated urinary 5-H1AA and plasma chromogranin
- Octreotide can be used in treatment.

References

1 Gage BF, van Walraven C, Pearce L, *et al.* Selecting patients with atrial fibrillation for anticoagulation: stroke risk stratification in patients taking aspirin. *Circulation.* 2004; **110** (16): 2287–92.

2 British Thoracic Society and SIGN. *British Guideline on the Management of Asthma. A national clinical guideline.* Revised ed. London: BTS; 2009.

3 British Thoracic Society. *The Management of Community Acquired Pneumonia in Adults.* London: BTS; 2004.

4 Henry M, Arnold T, Harvey J, on behalf of the British Thoracic Society Pleural Disease Group, a subgroup of the British Thoracic Society Standards of Care Committee. BTS Guidelines for the Management of Spontaneous Pneumothorax. *Thorax.* 2003; **58**.

5 National Institute for Health and Clinical Excellence. *Management of Type 2 Diabetes – management of blood pressure and blood lipids (Guideline H).* London: NICE; 2002.

Bibliography

- Kalra PA. *Essential Revision Notes for MRCP*. Revised ed. PasTest; 2003.
- Longmore M, Wilkinson I, Rajagopalan S. *Oxford Handbook of Clinical Medicine*. 6th ed. Oxford: Oxford University Press; 2004.
- Bloom S, Webster G. *Oxford Handbook of Gastroenterolgy and Hepatology*. Oxford: Oxford University Press; 2006.
- Moore K, Dalley A. *Clinically Orientated Anatomy*. 4th ed. Canada: Lippincott Williams and Wilkins; 1999.
- Lote C. *Principles of Renal Physiology*. 4th ed. Boston: Kluwer Academic; 2000.
- Kumar P, Clark M. *Clinical Medicine*. 5th ed. London: W.B. Saunders; 2002.
- Stevens A, Lowe J. *Human Histology*. 2nd ed. London: Harcourt International; 1999.
- Bear M, Connors B, Paradiso M. *Neuroscience: exploring the brain*. 2nd ed. USA: Lippincott Williams and Wilkins; 2001.
- Crossman AR, Neary D. *Neuroanatomy: an illustrated colour text*. 2nd ed. London: Harcourt; 2000.
- Munro J, Campell I. *Macleods Clinical Examination*. 10th ed. London: Elsevier; 2000.